Introduction to Clinical

Introduction to Clinical Examination

John F. Munro MB ChB (Hons) FRCPE

Consultant Physician, Eastern General and Edenhall Hospitals, Edinburgh;
Part-time Senior Lecturer, Faculty of Medicine, Edinburgh University

Michael J. Ford MB ChB MD FRCPE

Consultant Physician, Eastern General and Leith Hospitals, Edinburgh;
Member of the Clinical Teaching Staff, Faculty of Medicine,
Edinburgh University

FIFTH EDITION

CHURCHILL LIVINGSTONE
EDINBURGH LONDON MELBOURNE AND NEW YORK 1989

CHURCHILL LIVINGSTONE
Medical Division of Longman Group UK Limited

Distributed in the United States of America by Churchill Livingstone Inc.,
1560 Broadway, New York, N.Y. 10036, and by associated companies,
branches and representatives throughout the world.

First edition 1974   Fourth edition 1985
Second edition 1977   Fifth edition 1989
Third edition 1983   Reprinted 1990

ISBN 0-443-04078-8

British Library Cataloguing in Publication Data
Introduction to clinical examination. — 5th ed.
  1. Man. Diagnosis. Physical examination
  I. Munro, J F (John Forbes), 1933– II. Ford,
  Michael J (Michael Joseph) 1949
  616.07'54

Library of Congress Cataloging in Publication Data
Munro, J. F. (John Forbes)
    Introduction to clinical examination/John F. Munro, Michael J.
Ford. — 5th ed.
      p.   cm.
    Fifth ed. of: Introduction to clinical examination/John Macleod,
E. B. French, J. F. Munro. 4th ed. 1985.
    Bibliography: p.
    Includes index.
    1. Physical diagnosis.   I. Ford, Michael J.   II. Macleod, John.
Introduction to clinical examination.   III. Title.
RC76.M865   1989   88-38905
616.07'54—dc19   CIP

Produced by Longman Singapore Publishers (Pte) Ltd.
Printed in Singapore

Preface

This pocketbook aims to provide the junior medical student with a brief account of the fundamental methods of clinical examination. It is intended to be of service at the outset of clinical training, at a stage when many students feel overwhelmed by detail. Senior students have also found the book to be an effective aid for revision.

Guidance is first provided about history-taking and attention is directed to the principal symptoms of disease of the main systems. The basic techniques of physical examination are then described; the simple instruction given about these should augment the teaching provided by clinical tutors and make it easier to learn from observing experienced practitioners at work. Most of the methods can be developed by practice on colleagues so that some proficiency and self-reliance can be acquired before the student examines patients. Only brief reference is made to the significance of the physical findings and mention of diseases is confined to those which are commonly encountered or illustrate a specific point. A simple system of case-recording is also included at the end of the book.

Skills, once acquired, improve with practice; meanwhile the assessment of clinical data in terms of basic science must be studied. Such information and an introduction to further investigation are available in *Clinical Examination* 7th edition 1986, edited by Macleod and Munro, and published by

Churchill Livingstone. The reading of a more advanced text-book of this type will be more meaningful after a few months of clinical experience. Then the emphasis can be changed from 'how' to 'why'—from the methods of data collection to their interpretation and, with that, the cultivation of critical judgment and independent thought.

Edinburgh, 1989   J.F.M.
                                                                     M.J.F.

Acknowledgements

The editors wish to thank past and present authors of the parent textbook *Clinical Examination*, particularly Drs I W B Grant, M B Matthews and the late Clifford Mawdsley, Mr J H S Scott and Professors J A Strong and H J Walton, who generously allowed us to adapt their original contributions.

The editors are also grateful to many others who have given assistance and constructive criticisms. They wish to thank Ian Hughes for producing the artwork. Finally, they are very deeply indebted to Dr John Macleod and Dr E B French for their enormous editorial contributions to previous editions of this book and for their continuing support of the present edition.

Contents

1. The approach to the patient

THE HISTORY

The history is the patient's account of the illness and is often
the most important part of the clinical assessment. It de-
scribes current problems, enables the clinician to obtain an
initial appraisal of the patient's personality and points to
where particular emphasis should be laid during the physical
examination. In taking a history there are three main stages.
The first is a brief introduction. The second is the principal
stage during which the doctor listens carefully to the patient's
story. The third is an interrogation by the doctor to clarify
the foregoing and to extract further information about the
present symptoms, previous health, family history and the
social setting. The student should practise a routine in these
three stages. As experience is acquired, the sequence and
emphasis can be adapted to contend with any clinical situation. In other words, a methodical but flexible approach is
the fundamental skill in obtaining a history.

Stage 1: The introduction

Students, like doctors, should introduce themselves by name
and give a friendly greeting. They should ask for, and
remember, the patient's name. Most patients welcome
students whom they regard as members of the medical team;

1

some may be tired of being questioned or examined and others may be depressed because they are ill or apprehensive in a strange environment. If there are difficulties in establishing a satisfactory relationship, the student should try to determine the reason and if in doubt, consult with the medical or nursing staff. An introductory chat about impersonal matters may help the patient to adapt to yet another stranger. For example, conversation about the patient's occupation can often initiate good rapport. From the outset, students should learn to acquire a professional attitude, detached but not uncaring. They must learn to be patient, particularly with the elderly and the deaf, and not to react to troublesome patients with criticism, anger or dismissal. They must also recognise that some individuals will try to manipulate them, for example by flattery, inviting opinions about diagnosis or treatment; such enquiries should be referred to the medical staff. The student can learn much about the complex interactions between patient and doctor by attempting to analyse unusual feelings aroused by patients and discussing problems of this type with a tutor.

Stage 2: The patient's account of the current illness

The patient should now be prompted to speak about current problems by an opening remark such as: 'Please tell me about your present trouble' or 'When were you last quite well?' followered by 'What has happened since?' Students must learn to be good listeners and not be too eager to ask questions. The patient must be encouraged to continue the story right up to the time of interview. When given the opportunity many patients will provide much information about their illness and themselves. They often need to talk about their troubles and clinicians who recognise this and provide an understanding audience usually establish a good relationship quickly. It is not difficult for students to acquire this skill. While premature interruption should be avoided, occasionally it is necessary to steer the loquacious individual from irrelevant detail or to help the inarticulate patient by posing simple questions. Sometimes information is suppressed involuntarily because of anxiety or fear of disease such as cancer, but occasionally the patient may deliberately mislead the doctor. This happens notably in alcoholics and other drug abusers or addicts. It may also be a feature of some patients with severe personality disorders. In such cases critical listening will often detect inconsistencies.

Some patients may be unable to give a history because they are too acutely ill, confused, demented or unconscious. In such circumstances as much information as possible should be obtained from a relative or neighbour, and the general practitioner.

Stage 3: Interrogation

When the patient has completed the account of the current illness, the next step is to clarify the description by specific questioning and to obtain a chronological account of the development of the illness from the first symptom to the time of interview. Precise dates are to be preferred to vague statements such as 'a short while ago'. It may be necessary to obtain more detail about certain symptoms; for example, the *analysis of pain* is based upon data about the following 10 features:

1. Main site	6. Frequency and periodicity
2. Radiation	7. Special times of occurrence
3. Character	8. Aggravating factors
4. Severity	9. Relieving factors
5. Duration	10. Associated phenomena.

Questions should be simple and without bias but the history will be misleading if the patient's interpretations are accepted uncritically; for example, 'flu' or 'rheumatism' may really be serious disease. It is often of value to find out which investigations and treatments have been performed and what the patient has been told about the present illness.

When the history has been clarified by answers to specific questions about presenting problems, enquiry should be made about other systems, drugs, allergies, previous illness and the family and social background.

Systemic enquiry

Significant symptoms may not be mentioned because of embarrassment or because they appear unimportant to the patient. Questions should therefore be asked about principal symptoms concerning the major systems, such as breathlessness, cough, pain, headache, visual impairment, indigestion (the imprecise word being used deliberately to broaden the scope), bowel, urinary or menstrual troubles and changes in appetite, weight and sleep.

Drugs and allergies

It is essential to know about the patient's medication, as any drug may cause ill effects. Some, such as anticoagulants or corticosteroids, are potentially so dangerous that the patient should carry a card giving details of the treatment. Past medication can also be hazardous. For example aspirin containing compounds may cause gastrointestinal haemorrhage. Such dangers may be overlooked if the necessary enquiry is not made. If there is doubt, it may be necessary to ask the patient to produce pills for identification. Any allergy should be recorded in a conspicuous position on the patient's notes.

Previous illness, state of health and foreign travel

In addition to a list of previous illnesses, it is also helpful to know about the outcome of any medical or radiological examination carried out for employment or insurance purposes. It is also necessary to know about any travel or residence abroad, as infectious disease can readily be imported. Among many possible tropical diseases, the recognition of falciparum malaria is most important if fatalities are to be avoided. When confronted with an illness where the cause is not immediately obvious, it is vital to ask, 'Have you ever been abroad?'

Family history

The frequency of inherited and environmental factors in the aetiology of disease makes it essential to know about the age and health, or cause of death of the patient's parents, spouse, siblings and other close relatives. A method of recording the family history is shown in Figure 1 and illustrated by an inherited disorder.

Social and personal history

An individual's health and well-being are affected by occupational, social and personal factors. In hospital the student sees the patient in an artificial setting. Knowledge of the individual's background is necessary not only for diagnosis but also for management. How patients live, think and behave will influence how they cope with illness. It is important to obtain details of the patient's lifestyle and personal relationships. Enquiry should therefore be made about such factors as employment status, housing, personal relationships (or lack of them), leisure interests, physical exercise and the use of drugs including alcohol and tobacco.

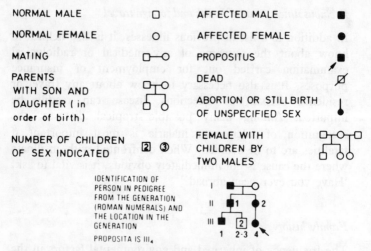

Fig. 1 Symbols used in pedigree charts. Drawing up a family tree beginning with the affected person first found to have the trait (propositus if male, proposita if female). Thereafter relevant information regarding siblings and all maternal and paternal relatives is included. (Adapted from *Elements of Medical Genetics*, by A E H Emery. Churchill Livingstone, Edinburgh, 1982)

Male subjects consuming more than 30 gms of alcohol (3 units per day are at risk of developing an alcohol-related disorder. The risk in females occurs if the daily intake exceeds 20 gms (2 units).

THE PSYCHOLOGICAL ASSESSMENT

In every illness it is necessary to evaluate the relevant psychological factors. The account of the history and the manner in which it is delivered usually reveal much about the patient's personality and emotional state. A patient who becomes upset at any stage of the proceedings should be encouraged to talk, as this may reveal a problem such as an unsatisfactory personal relationship or a bereavement. When it becomes apparent that the patient has a psychological difficulty, a psychiatric assessment is indicated. This comprises three basic elements: a psychiatric history, an examination of the mental state and an evaluation of the personality.

1. The psychiatric history

The history should be taken in a private and comfortable setting. The interviewer encourages the patient to speak about personal experiences, and acts as a guide rather than an interrogator; the question and answer technique is inappropriate because that approach does not leave patients free to introduce their own concerns. Sensitive subjects such as sex or bereavement, should be discussed frankly and directly. Accounts of unusual behaviour should be broached without equivocation. For example such enquiry may be welcomed by a depressed patient as a much needed opportunity to disclose painful impulses towards suicide. A detailed chronological account of the patient's life is not required. Instead the interviewer collates information as it emerges about the present illness, the relationships the patient has with each parent and sibling, the adaptation made to schooling and to puberty, adolescent friendships, the development of independence, employment, courtship, marriage and about attitudes towards spouse and children. Gaps can be filled by specific enquiry towards the end of the interview.

2. Examination of the mental state

Certain features may have become apparent in the course of the history which will indicate where further exploration is required; for example, a vague or contradictory history may be due to intellectual impairment. Some or all of the following aspects may require to be assessed:

General appearance and behaviour

The patient's expression, clothes, mannerisms and reactions to the clinician, should be described briefly.

Thought processes

Talk is externalised thought and indicates how the patient arranges and expresses concepts. A sample of talk should be recorded.

Mood (affect)

Information about the prevailing affect will have been obtained in the earlier stages of the examination. It may be necessary to supplement this by specific enquiry such as: 'What is your mood like?', 'Do you worry or get depressed?' and 'Do you have any difficulties sleeping?'

Delusions, hallucinations and obsessions

Patients may reveal in their talk that they harbour false beliefs, or experience sensory impressions without corresponding sensory stimuli or are preoccupied by persistent obtrusive thoughts.

Intellectual functions

Acute or chronic brain impairment leads respectively to temporary or permanent deterioration of intellectual functions. This part of the examination requires evaluation as follows:

(i) *Orientation* in time and place can be assessed by asking the year, the month, the day of the week, and the time and place of interview.

(ii) *Memory* is tested by the patient's ability to recall both remote and recent events.

(iii) *Attention and concentration.* The patient may be preoccupied or distracted and be unable to pay attention during the interview. Concentration can be tested by the '*serial sevens*' test. The patient is asked to substract 7 from 100 and to continue to take 7 from the remainder. Most people complete the test within one minute and make no more than two mistakes.

(iv) *General information* is tested by asking questions about current affairs, e.g. national politics and international problems.

(v) *Intelligence* is assessed from patients' accounts of themselves, their occupation and extent of their knowledge; their capacity to reason can be judged by asking them to explain the meaning of proverbs.

Intelligence can also be measured by the use of standardised tests—the normal Intelligence Quotient (IQ) range is 80 to 120.

3. Evaluation of the personality

After the psychiatric history and the examination of the mental state the interviewer should be able to make an assessment of the patient's personality and recognise excessive dependency on others, hysterical or obsessive traits, or schizoid tendencies characterised by an unusual aloofness. Thus a serious social maladaptation such as excessive hostility towards other people may be identified.

Conclusions on completion of the history

The history should suggest the diagnosis, or at least a differential diagnosis in most cases, and thus direct the student to make a thorough examination appropriate to the diagnostic probabilities.

THE PHYSICAL EXAMINATION—GENERAL PRINCIPLES

Privacy and warmth are essential; in a hospital ward or out-patient department, screens must be drawn round the bed or couch before the examination begins. An adjustable back rest is essential for the dyspnoeic patient who becomes more breathless when lying flat. Illumination must be good; exposure of the area to be examined must be adequate but not to an extent that might unnecessarily embarrass or chill the patient. Both patient and the examiner must be warm; apart from the discomfort, shivering causes muscle sounds which interfere with auscultation, while abdominal palpation with cold hands will cause the muscles to contract and impair the efficiency of the examination. Much of the clinical examination is best conducted from the patient's right side. It is imperative that the handling of any painful area is gentle. While students should take every opportunity to conduct as comprehensive an examination as is acceptable to the patient, exhaustion as the result of prolonged examination must be avoided; the risk of this is greatest in the frail or elderly. Apprehensive female patients require special consideration by the young male student. There is usually no difficulty in a hospital ward, but if the student has any doubts, the medical or nursing staff should be consulted.

At the conclusion of the examination the findings should be recorded systematically (p. 128). Diagrams should be used to define the site and extent of physical findings such as swellings (p. 116) or the effects of trauma. The student should learn first how to collect and record the facts, identify the patient's problems and then, possibly with the help of a tutor, decide on a management plan. This may involve further investigations before a diagnosis is established and treatment initiated.

THE SEQUENCE OF THE LEARNING PROCESS

1. Practise history taking from the outset using the guidelines given in this chapter.

2. Through reading and clinical teaching and by observing experts, acquire the techniques for the examination of one system at a time. Then preferably practise on a colleague before examining a patient.

3. During the history and while examining individual systems, learn to observe general features such as the patient's demeanour, or local changes such as skin lesions, and note them for elucidation later.

4. Towards the end of the first clinical term, learn to integrate techniques along the lines described in Chapter 7 so that the examination is conducted with a minimum of inconvenience to the patient.

2. The cardiovascular system

THE HISTORY

1. Symptoms of cardiac disease

The principal symptoms are retrosternal pain, breathlessness, oedema of the dependent parts and palpitation.

Pain is most commonly due to myocardial ischaemia. Angina pectoris is characteristically brought on by an increase in cardiac work as induced by exercise or sudden emotion. It is relieved by rest within a few minutes. In contrast, the pain of myocardial infarction may commence when the patient is at rest and persist. Cardiac pain should be analysed as outlined on page 3. The main site is usually retrosternal where the pain may be described as 'a tightness', often attributed by the patient to 'indigestion'. Radiation commonly occurs to the left shoulder and arm, but the pain may be felt in either or both arms, the neck, jaws, back and sometimes the epigastrium. The pain of myocardial infarction may be accompanied by breathlessness, nausea, sweating and a sensation of impending doom (angor animi).

Breathlessness occurring on exertion and relieved by rest is usually the earliest symptom of left heart failure. It is due to decreased lung compliance caused initially by pulmonary venous congestion. Sometimes the patient may be wakened from sleep by dyspnoea due to acute pulmonary oedema and be forced to sit up to obtain relief. This *paroxysmal nocturnal dyspnoea* may be accompanied by cough and sometimes by the production of watery sputum which may be blood-stained. If breathlessness is persistent, the patient is compelled to sit upright to obtain relief; this is known as *orthopnoea*.

Dependent oedema of cardiac origin is due to the adverse effects of cardiac failure on renal function causing salt and water retention. Its' distribution is directly proportional to the capillary pressures and it is most marked in dependent areas.

Palpitation is an awareness of the heart beat. This can be caused by fright, anxiety, ectopic beats or arrhythmias.

The patient should be asked to illustrate the frequency and rhythm by tapping a finger on the chest.

Syncope, or the sensation of sudden faintness without actual loss of consciousness, may be cardiac in origin; for example secondary to a cardiac arrhythmia.

2. Symptoms of arterial disease

Ischaemia due to severe atheroma leads to symptoms which are determined by the area supplied. Three clinical pictures are commonly seen:

  (i) In the heart, angina pectoris or myocardial infarction occurs.
 (ii) In the legs, pain in the calf on walking causes limping (*intermittent claudication*) and the patient may have to stop until the pain is relieved by rest. Sometimes distal gangrene may develop.
(iii) In the brain, hemiplegia or other neurological defects arise.

Acute arterial occlusion of an organ or limb may be the result of an embolus from the left side of the heart.

3. Symptoms of venous disease

Thrombosis of a major vein in the leg may cause local pain with redness, warmth, swelling and tenderness of the leg. However major venous thrombosis may remain undetected until the advent of pulmonary embolus or infarction causes such symptoms as collapse, breathlessness, pleural pain or haemoptysis.

THE PHYSICAL EXAMINATION

This should start with a general inspection of the patient, particular attention being paid to breathlessness and cyanosis. The radial arterial and jugular venous pulses are studied next. The heart is then examined by inspection, palpation and auscultation. The blood pressure is usually recorded at the end of the examination in the hope that the patient will be more relaxed. Signs of cardiac failure in other systems are sought when the lungs, liver, trunk and legs are examined. Inspection of the fundus oculi for arterial changes, haemorrhages, exudates and papilloedema is particularly relevant in arterial hypertension.

The arterial pulse

The radial pulse is examined at the wrist with regard to the rate, rhythm, form of the pulse wave, volume and state of the vessel wall.

Rate

The adult average of 72 beats per minute (range 50–100) is exceeded in children or in response to exercise, anxiety, fever or hyperthyroidism. Rates at rest of 40 or less may be due to heart block, and of more than 120 may be due to ectopic foci becoming 'pacemakers' as in paroxysmal tachycardia.

Rhythm

This is normally regular though, especially in the young, the rate may quicken on inspiration (sinus arrhythmia). Irregular rhythm is most commonly due to ectopic beats or atrial fibrillation.

Form of the pulse wave

The wave may rise more suddenly than normal when diastolic pressure is low and the systolic well maintained. The resultant slapping sensation is increased by raising the arm (and decreased by lowering it) due to the hydrostatic effect upon the blood pressure. This 'collapsing pulse' is most striking in severe aortic incompetence. By contrast a prolonged wave of low amplitude is characteristic of stenosis of the aortic valve.

Volume

Providing that the form of the pulse wave and the calibre and elasticity of the artery are normal, the size of the wave is proportional to left ventricular stroke volume.

Vessel wall

Hardening and tortuosity are usually due to Mönckeberg's medial sclerosis, a non-occlusive arterial disease of little importance, commonly found in the elderly.

The blood pressure

The patient should be sitting or lying comfortably and relaxed, for anxiety raises the blood pressure. An inflatable rubber bag contained in a cuff is placed with its centre over the brachial artery and the cuff wound smoothly and firmly

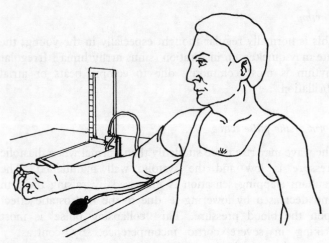

Fig. 2   Measurement of the blood pressure.

around the arm (see Fig. 2). The systolic pressure is that required to obliterate the radial pulse. The brachial pulse is then located and the cuff reinflated to just over systolic pressure. Auscultation over the brachial artery as the pressure is reduced gives the systolic pressure when Korotkov sounds are first heard; the diastolic pressure is when these sounds become muffled or disappear.

Jugular venous pressure

This is measured as the vertical height of the peak of the internal jugular venous pulse above the manubriosternal angle (Fig. 3); it can be roughly estimated in cm of blood if it is assumed that one finger's breadth is approximately 2 cm. Normally the venous pressure is less than 3 cm and thus in a healthy person reclining with the trunk at 45° from the horizontal, the jugular venous pulse should not be seen above the level of the clavicle. It falls during inspiration. Pressure

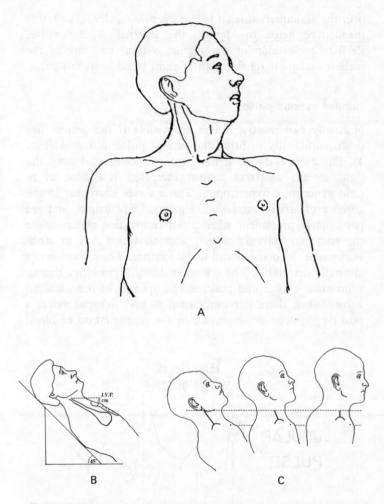

Fig. 3 Estimation of the jugular venous pressure. The observer is looking for the uppermost point of distension of the right internal jugular vein deep to the sternomastoid muscle. In cardiac failure, the central venous pressure is visible above the level of the clavicle whatever the position of the patient. (C) shows effect of position on a raised jugular venous pressure.

over the abdomen causes it to rise (*'hepato-jugular reflux'*); this manoeuvre helps to identify the internal jugular pulse. Persistent elevation of the jugular venous pressure is the earliest and most reliable sign of right sided heart failure.

Jugular venous pulse

Normally two positive waves are visible if the patient lies down sufficiently to bring the venous pulse into view (Fig. 4). The *a* wave, due to atrial systole, is exaggerated when the right atrium contracts against increased resistance as in right ventricular hypertrophy. The *a* waves disappear in the absence of atrial contraction, e.g. atrial fibrillation, and are particularly prominent when atrial contraction occurs while the tricuspid valve is closed, 'cannon waves', as in atrio-ventricular dissociation and nodal rhythm. The *c* wave is not clinically detectable. The *v* wave is due to atrial filling during ventricular systole and peaks at the opening of the tricuspid valve. When there is regurgitation at the tricuspid valve, a positive, systolic *cv* wave due to the regurgitation of blood

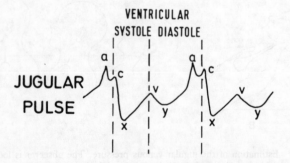

Fig. 4 Form of the venous pulse wave, a = atrial systole; c = onset of ventricular systole; v = peak pressure in right atrium at opening of tricuspid valve; a − x = x descent, due to atrial relaxation; v − y = y descent at commencement of ventricular filling.

into the atrium replaces the usual dip in pressure in early systole.

The carotid pulse can be distinguished from the normal venous pulse as the former is readily palpable and does not alter with the position of the patient or with pressure on the abdomen.

THE EXAMINATION OF THE HEART

Inspection

The patient should be semirecumbent and relaxed with the head comfortably supported. The examiner notes any asymmetry of the chest wall which may have displaced the heart. The precordium is then inspected for the site of the apical impulse and other pulsations, including a left parasternal movement due to right ventricular hypertrophy and a pulsation in the second left intercostal space arising from an enlarged pulmonary artery. Retraction or pulsation is often seen high in the epigastrium due respectively to contraction of the heart or expansion of the abdominal aorta.

Palpation

The precordium is palpated for normal and abnormal pulsations and for thrills. The examiner attempts to localize the *apex beat* by placing the right hand on the left chest wall. The apex beat is the furthest point downwards and outwards on the chest wall where the finger can feel the apical impulse. It is normally in the fifth intercostal space and medial to the midclavicular line. Sometimes, particularly in a patient with a thick chest wall or emphysema, the apical impulse is impalpable. It may be displaced by deformity of the chest wall or spine, by diseases of the lungs or pleura, or by cardiac enlargement. The apical impulse is abnormally forceful in left ventricular hypertrophy and is 'heaving' or 'thrusting' in

character, whereas a 'tapping' sensation is felt in mitral stenosis due to abnormal closure of the mitral valve.

Palpation of the rest of the precordium may reveal a left
lower parasternal lift due to right ventricular hypertrophy or
some other abnormal movement. A murmur may be so loud
as to be palpable as a *thrill* which is a vibrating sensation.
Thrills arising at the mitral valve are best felt at the apex with
the patient lying on the left side. Other thrills are most
readily detected when the patient leans forward with the
breath held in expiration.

Auscultation

A stethoscope with both a bell and a diaphragm should be
used. The bell placed lightly on the skin is better for the
detection of low-pitched sounds whereas high-pitched sounds
are best heard through the diaphragm pressed firmly against
the skin. The ear pieces must fit comfortably and the spring

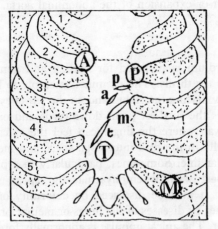

Fig. 5 Position of the heart valves and auscultatory areas

should be strong enough to hold them firmly in place. The tubing should be about 25 cm in length and thick enough to reduce external noise.

Auscultation should be carried out all over the precordium and the great vessels. Many clinicians listen first to the apex but it may be preferable to start in the second left intercostal space where the two components of the normal second heart sound are the best heard (Fig. 5). This provides a reliable point of orientation in the cardiac cycle. After listening to the first and second heart sounds and the intervals between them, the following questions should be posed:

1. Are the first and second sounds normal?
2. Are there any added sounds?
3. Are there any murmurs?

1. The heart sounds

Attention should be paid to the quality of the heart sounds, their relative and absolute intensity and the presence or absence of splitting.

The normal *first heart sound* is loudest at the apex and is mainly due to closure of the mitral valve, the tricuspid component being minor. The intensity is reduced in mitral regurgitation and increased in the presence of mitral stenosis where its quality is more abrupt in keeping with the tapping apical impulse. The first sound varies in intensity in the presence of an irregular rhythm or complete heart block.

The normal *second heart sound* is best heard at the left sternal edge in the second intercostal space. It is caused by closure of the aortic and pulmonary valves. During inspiration closure of the pulmonary valve is delayed, producing the normal physiological splitting. Any process which further delays closure will accentuate this splitting, e.g. pulmonary hypertension or right bundle branch block.

2. Added sounds

The *third heart sound*, commonly heard at the apex in healthy children and young adults, occurs during early ventricular filling and is low-pitched. When audible in older people it is usually indicative of heart failure. It is a feature of mitral incompetence.

The *fourth heart sound* is coincident with atrial contraction and thus precedes the first heart sound. It is low-pitched and indicative of atrial hypertrophy. It may occur in systemic hypertension.

Gallop rhythm is a term sometimes used to describe the existence of tachycardia with a triple rhythm due to a third or fourth heart sound or a summation of both.

An *opening snap* of the mitral valve is pathognomonic of mitral stenosis and occurs soon after the second sound. It is clicking in quality and best heard between the apex and the left sternal edge.

Pericardial friction is the characteristic sign of pericarditis. It is usually best heard with the diaphragm pressed firmly against the chest, often to the left of the lower end of the sternum. It is a creaking or rustling noise often with three components in each cardiac cycle, sounding like 'chi-te-chi'.

3. Murmurs

Murmurs arise from turbulent blood flow and may occur if a valve is diseased or if a large amount of blood flows through a normal valve. The characteristics of any murmur should be noted in respect of site, radiation, pitch, timing and intensity.

Site. The area over which a murmur is best heard depends upon the valve of origin or cardiac defect and the direction of the blood flow (Fig. 5). Mitral murmurs are best heard at the apex and ejection murmurs arising at the aortic valve are often maximal in the second intercostal space to the right of the sternal edge (Fig. 6).

Radiation occurs along the line of blood flow. It follows that mid-systolic (ejection) aortic murmurs radiate into the neck and aortic regurgitant murmurs down the left sternal edge; they may sometimes be best heard at the sites to which they are transmitted (Fig. 6).

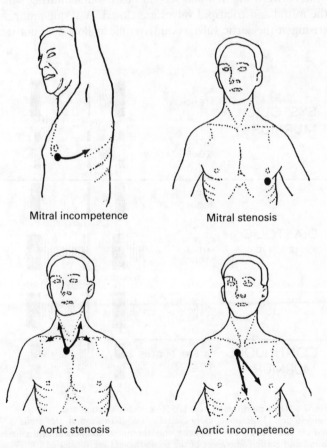

Mitral incompetence   Mitral stenosis

Aortic stenosis   Aortic incompetence

Fig. 6 Areas of maximum intensity and selective radiation.

Pitch may be characteristic. Thus the murmur of mitral stenosis is low-pitched, whereas that of aortic regurgitation is high-pitched.

Timing. Murmurs are usually systolic or diastolic, but rarely may be both, e.g. the continuous murmur of a persistent ductus arteriosus (Fig. 7). Clinical systole is the time between the first and second heart sounds during which the mitral and tricuspid valves are closed. A systolic murmur arising at the aortic valve is mid-systolic as flow does not start

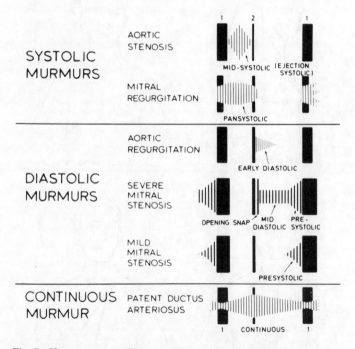

Fig. 7 Heart murmurs. These are (1) systolic (ejection and pansystolic), (2) diastolic (early diastolic, mid-diastolic and presystolic), and (3) continuous. For simplicity only the mitral component of the first sound and aortic component of the second sound are illustrated.

until ventricular pressure reaches aortic diastolic pressure; it then increases and finally tapers off before the aortic valve closes to cause a 'diamond shaped' ejection systolic murmur. The mitral regurgitant murmur continues throughout systole producing a pansystolic murmur that may obscure the first and second heart sounds.

Clinical diastole, which comprises the time between the second and the first heart sounds, can be divided into three phases. Early diastole extends from the closing of the aortic and pulmonary valves to the opening of the mitral and tricuspid valves. In mid-diastole, passive filling of the ventricles occurs; presystole comprises atrial systole up to the closing of the mitral and tricuspid valves. It follows that aortic regurgitant murmurs will commence in early diastole whereas the murmur of mitral stenosis commences in mid-diastole and is accentuated by atrial contraction during presystole. Sometimes only the presystolic component can be heard in mitral stenosis, but if there is atrial fibrillation, presystolic accentuation does not occur. Comparable murmurs arise less commonly in the right side of the heart.

Murmurs are best timed in relation to the first and second heart sounds. Heart sounds are usually better heard at the base of the heart. The first heart sound can be identified by its coincidence with the apical impulse; if this cannot be felt, then the carotid pulse may be used to time a murmur. The radial pulse is unsuitable as it is delayed by about 0.15 secs.

A mitral diastolic murmur is best heard with the bell chestpiece lightly applied at the apex with the patient half-turned on to the left side and it may become louder immediately after some exercise. The diastolic murmur of aortic regurgitation is best heard with the diaphragm firmly applied along the left lower sternal edge while the patient leans forward with the breath held in expiration.

Intensity of a murmur may be graded as follows:

Grade 1: Just audible by an expert in optimal conditions

Grade 2: Quiet; just audible by a student in optimal conditions

Grade 3: Moderately loud

Grade 4: Loud

Grade 5: Very loud ⎫ accompanied by

Grade 6: Audible without stethoscope ⎭ a thrill

Signs of cardiac failure

These must be sought by inspecting the J.V.P. (p. 16), by palpating the abdomen for enlargement and tenderness of the liver (p. 52), auscultating the lungs for crepitations (p. 44) and testing for dependent pitting oedema (p. 116).

THE EXAMINATION OF PERIPHERAL ARTERIES

Acute arterial insufficiency of a limb leads to pain, weakness and sensory impairment, coldness, pallor or cyanosis and maybe to gangrene. Chronic ischaemia also causes pain (intermittent claudication, p. 13) and nutritional changes. Manifestations of the latter are failure of growth of nails, loss of hairs and atrophy of subcutaneous tissues of the digits.

Comparison should be made of the two limbs. The legs are far more commonly affected than the arms. Signs of arterial insufficiency will be greatest at the periphery. Inspection, palpation and auscultation are the methods employed.

Inspection

The two limbs are compared for pallor and cyanosis and for evidence of nutritional changes.

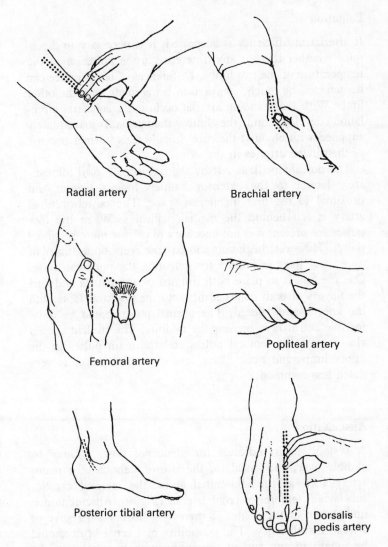

Radial artery

Brachial artery

Femoral artery

Popliteal artery

Posterior tibial artery

Dorsalis pedis artery

Fig. 8 Palpation of peripheral pulses.

Palpation

If arterial insufficiency is suspected, it is necessary to determine whether there is any difference in the pulses or in the temperature of the two limbs. Differences of temperature can be detected by touch, comparison being made with the other limb. With longstanding arterial occlusion a collateral circulation develops and the limb, though still inadequately supplied with blood at the core, usually feels warmer because of the dilated arteries in the skin.

The dorsalis pedis is felt by the fingertips placed immediately lateral to the extensor hallucis longus tendon and proximal to the first metatarsal space. The posterior tibial artery is felt behind the medial malleolus. When the foot pulses are present it is not necessary to palpate more proximal pulses. However, beginners should take every opportunity of improving their technique for palpating the popliteal pulse. One method is to place both thumbs on the patella and curl the fingers of both hands firmly into the popliteal fossa with the knee slightly flexed. The normal pulse should be quite forcible and it is in or near the midline. The student should also palpate the femoral pulses and the main pulses in the upper limbs and neck where loss of arterial pulses is very much less common.

Auscultation

A systolic bruit indicates turbulence of flow. It may be audible over, and distal to, the site of stenosis of a major artery such as the abdominal aorta, the internal carotid, subclavian, femoral or renal arteries (Fig. 9). Auscultation is undertaken at these sites if there is a history suggestive of arterial insufficiency. The possibility of a renal bruit should be sought in any patient presenting with hypertension. An aortic bruit is sometimes present in a healthy subject.

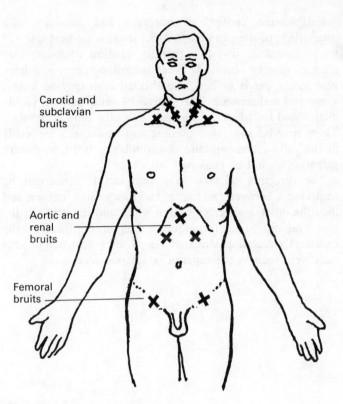

Carotid and
subclavian
bruits

Aortic and
renal
bruits

Femoral
bruits

Fig. 9   Sites of major arterial bruits.

THE EXAMINATION OF PERIPHERAL VEINS

Inflammation or thrombosis of a vein may cause local discomfort or pain but extensive thrombus can be present and yet not cause symptoms. The clinical manifestations of venous obstruction depend on its site and extent together with the adequacy of collateral vessels. Distal to the obstruction there may be distension of the veins, cyanosis and oedema.

Examination consists of *inspection* and *palpation* with comparison of the two limbs. Varicose veins are best assessed when distended by the patient standing. Inflammatory changes may be observed. When occlusion occurs in a large vein in the pelvis or legs, the affected limb may be larger, shiny and oedematous. The superficial veins may be visibly dilated and fail to empty normally when the limb is elevated. There may be associated swelling and tenderness, especially in the calf, a common site of thrombosis, but unnecessary palpation should be avoided.

The direction of flow in a vein can be discerned by emptying it between two fingers and then raising first one and then the other to determine from which end the vein fills the more rapidly. This technique is helpful in assessing the collateral circulation which develops after obstruction of a main vein such as the superior or inferior vena cava.

3. The respiratory system

THE HISTORY

The principal symptoms of respiratory disease are cough, sputum, haemoptysis, chest pain, dyspnoea, wheeze and stridor. Enquiry should also be made about symptoms caused by disease of the upper respiratory tract, such as nasal obstruction, bleeding and discharge, sore throat and hoarseness. Past and present tobacco smoking habits and any occupational hazard such as coal mining or exposure to asbestos should be noted.

Cough varies in nature depending on its cause. It may be harsh, dry and paroxysmal, loose and readily productive of sputum, or short and half-suppressed by pain.

Sputum may be mucoid (grey, white or 'clear'), purulent (yellow or green) or mucopurulent (a mixture of the two). If purulent, the amount of sputum produced may be of diagnosic importance, and the patient should be asked to estimate the daily volume.

Haemoptysis may range in amount from slight blood-staining of sputum to a massive haemorrhage. Frequently recurring haemoptysis, even of slight degree, is often of greater significance than a single episode.

Chest pain caused by pulmonary disease is characteristically unilateral and aggravated by deep inspiration and coughing ('pleuritic pain'). Although this is usually localised to the chest wall it is occasionally referred to the shoulder region ('diaphragmatic pain') or the anterior abdominal wall. Pain similar to that of pleurisy may be caused by disorders affecting the bones, muscles, nerves and joints of the chest wall and spine and by pericarditis.

Dyspnoea (shortness of breath) may be experienced only on exertion, or may occur in attacks when the patient is at rest. Non-respiratory causes of breathlessness include left heart failure, anaemia, obesity and anxiety.

Wheeze is a musical sound usually more conspicuous during expiration. It is almost invariably accompanied by dyspnoea and is due to obstruction of the small airways.

Stridor is a 'crowing' sound, produced in the larynx or trachea during inspiration and aggravated by coughing; it is due to obstruction of the large airways (larynx or trachea).

Further information about certain symptoms can be obtained from observation while the history is being recorded. Cough, for example, may lack its normal explosive character when a vocal cord is paralysed ('bovine' cough). A specimen of sputum should always be inspected, and hae-moptysis confirmed. Wheeze and stridor, which patients often find difficult to describe, can be recognised. Exertional breathlessness should be assessed by asking about exercise tolerance, for example 'how many flights of stairs can you climb without stopping?' Since dyspnoea is a subjective sensation, only the patient can be aware of it, but if breathing appears to be difficult and the cervical muscles are contracting during inspiration, it can be inferred that there is shortness of breath. Similarly, shallow breathing and half-suppressed coughing imply the presence of pleuritic pain.

Before proceeding to physical examination of the respir-atory system, it is important to look for finger clubbing (p. 109) and central cyanosis (p. 106), and to feel for enlarge-ment of the cervical lymph nodes, particularly those situated behind the clavicle in the region of the first rib ('scalene nodes'). (p. 113).

THE PHYSICAL EXAMINATION OF THE UPPER RESPIRATORY TRACT

It is possible by ordinary clinical methods to detect nasal obstruction and to inspect the mouth, teeth, pharynx and tonsils (p. 111). These observations should be made in every patient. Special equipment and expertise is required for the examination of the nasopharynx or larynx. Palpation of the trachea is described on page 36.

THE PHYSICAL EXAMINATION OF THE CHEST

Physical examination of the chest consists of inspection palpation, percussion and auscultation.

Inspection

The chest and upper abdomen should be fully exposed and evenly illuminated. Inspection is best undertaken with the patient standing or sitting. Minor asymmetry, which may be a guide to a major abnormality, may be seen better than when the patient is lying, as the chest movement is free. For access to the axillary areas, the palms of the patient's hands should rest behind or on top of the head. For optimal access to the back, the arms should be folded across the chest.

1. Lesions of the chest wall

Any abnormality should be inspected. Cutaneous or sub-cutaneous lesions, sub-cutaneous emphysema (recognised by a 'crackling' sensation on palpation), and localised deformities of the bones may require more detailed examination by palpation.

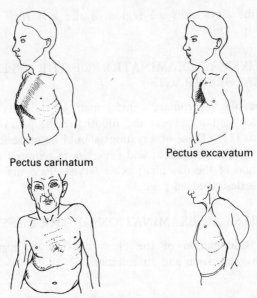

Pectus carinatum

Pectus excavatum

Thoracic kyphoscoliosis

Fig. 10 Chest wall deformities.

2. Abnormalities in the shape of the chest wall

In normal subjects the ratio of the anteroposterior diameter
of the chest relative to the lateral diameter is about 2 : 3.
These measurements may approximate in some patients with
emphysema (barrel chest) and in thoracic kyphosis (forward
curvature of the spine). *Pectus carinatum* (pigeon chest)
consists of a localised prominence of the sternum and adjacent
costal cartilages. It is often accompanied by indrawing of the
ribs to form symmetrical horizontal grooves (*Harrison's sulci*)
above everted costal margins and occurs as a sequel to child-
hood asthma and rickets. *Pectus excavatum* (funnel chest) is
a development defect in which there is a localised depression
of the lower end of the sternum or, less commonly,

depression of the whole length of the sternum and of the costal cartilages attached to it. This deformity may displace the heart but is usually asymptomatic. *Thoracic scoliosis* (lateral curvature of the spine) may alter the position of the mediastinum in relation to the anterior chest wall, with the result that abnormalities in the position of the trachea and the apex beat may be mistakenly attributed to cardiac or pulmonary disease (Fig. 10). Asymmetry is an important sign if scoliosis is not present as flattening implies underlying disease such as fibrosis or collapse of the lung.

3. *Study of respiratory movements*

(i) *Respiratory frequency* is counted unobtrusively. The normal rate is about 14 per minute in the adult.

(ii) *Respiratory depth* cannot be accurately measured by simple clinical assessment but it is possible to recognise marked degrees of hyper- or hypoventilation. The latter may be of considerable clinical importance in the diagnosis of ventilatory failure. Hyperventilation is due to stimulation of the respiratory centre as a result of anxiety, metabolic acidosis or head injury. Periodic or 'Cheyne Stokes' breathing is a cyclical variation in the depth of respiration, ranging from apnoea to hyperpnoea, due to decreased sensitivity of the respiratory centre to carbon dioxide. It occurs in left ventricular failure and brain stem ischaemia.

(iii) *Maximum chest expansion* is estimated by placing a tape measure round the chest at the level of the fourth or fifth costal cartilages and recording the maximum inspiratory/expiratory difference in the chest circumference. In the adult an expansion of less than 4 cm can be regarded as abnormal.

(iv) Observation of the *mode of breathing* can provide useful information. In normal subjects inspiration is mainly abdominal, effected by contraction of the diaphragm

and to a lesser extent thoracic. Chest expansion is
limited by pleurisy and contraction of the diaphragm is
reduced by peritonitis or abdominal distension.
Normal expiration is a passive process depending upon the
elastic recoil of the lungs.

(v) *Abnormal respiratory movements:*

    (a) Abnormal *inspiratory* movements. Generalised
indrawing of intercostal muscles occurs in patients
who cannot achieve adequate ventilation by normal
inspiratory efforts as, for example, when there is
gross hyper-inflation of the lungs in emphysema or
asthma.

        Local indrawing of a portion of the chest wall
during inspiration, 'paradoxical movement', occurs
in patients who have sustained double fractures of
a series of ribs or of the sternum and this may
produce severe respiratory distress.

    (b) Abnormal *expiratory* movements are produced by
powerful contractions of the abdominal muscles
and latissimus dorsi and are seen in asthma and
chronic bronchitis. Patients with severe airways
obstruction may also be seen to exhale by puffing
through pursed lips. This manoeuvre prevents
collapse of the bronchial walls and minimises the
work done during breathing.

(vi) *Asymmetry of movement.* Each side of the normal chest
moves symmetrically. Reduced movement affecting
part, or all, of one side is sometimes made more
obvious during a deep breath and when present is a
strong indication of underlying disease.

Palpation

The position of the mediastinum should be gauged by
palpating the trachea and locating the apex beat. The trachea

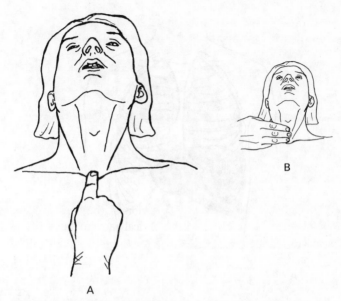

Fig. 11 A—identifying the position of the trachea; B—assessing the cricosternal distance.

should be felt by gently inserting the index finger tip into the suprasternal notch exactly in the midline and thereby detecting any deviation to one side or the other (Fig. 11). The distance between the cricoid cartilage and the suprasternal notch should also be noted as a reduction is a measure of the severity of obstructive airways disease.

Laying the hands gently on the pectoral regions below the clavicles often enables reduction in movement to be confirmed. Attention should be paid to both the duration and degree of movement. Similar observations should be made at the bases by laying the hands gently over each side of the chest. Grasping the chest must be avoided as it reduces the sensitivity of the test. A difference in movement may be more obvious on deep breathing (Fig. 13).

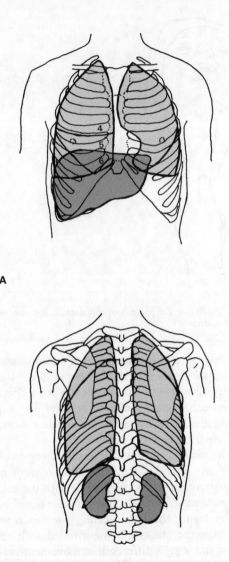

Fig. 12A   Surface anatomy of the viscera (anterior, posterior).

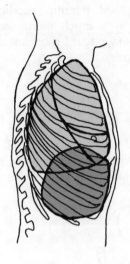

B

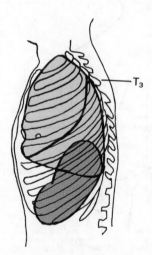

T₃

Fig. 12B Surface anatomy of the viscera (lateral).

Alterations in vocal fremitus parallel changes in vocal resonance which is a much more useful test (page 45). Vibration from a low pitched rhonchus or a pleural rub may sometimes be palpable.

Percussion

The *technique* is as follows:

1. A right-handed person places the left hand on the chest wall, palm downwards and with the fingers slightly separated, so that the second phalanx of the middle

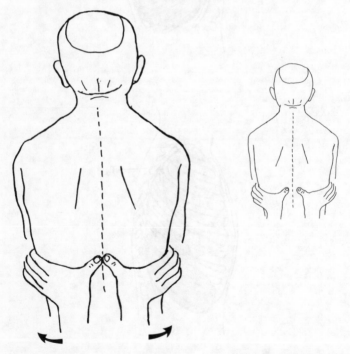

Fig. 13   Assessing respiratory movements of the lower ribs posteriorly.

finger is precisely over the area to be percussed. It is then pressed firmly against the chest wall, preferably along an intercostal space.

2. The centre of the second phalanx of the middle finger is struck sharply with the tip of the right middle finger. In order to produce a satisfactory percussion note the right middle finger must be held in a position of partial flexion, and the entire movement should come from the wrist joint (Fig. 14).

3. The note is compared over exactly equivalent areas of both lungs. When an area of altered resonance is discovered, its boundaries should be mapped out by percussing from a zone of normal resonance towards the suspected abnormality.

Percussion should be undertaken over the chest anteriorly, posteriorly and laterally. The apices of the upper lobes must not be overlooked (see Fig. 15). The subtle combination of change in pitch and duration of the percussion note can be learned only by experience, but an immediate impression of the value of the sign can be gained by comparing the note over the lung, the liver and the stomach.

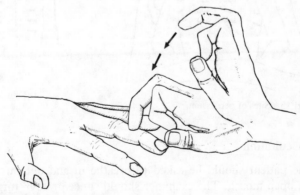

Fig. 14 Percussion technique.

Significance of changes in percussion note

The percussion note over normal lung is resonant. Resonance is impaired when the lung is separated from the chest wall by pleural fluid or thickening, or pulmonary consolidation or collapse. Over such lesions the percussion note is impaired or dull. A characteristic 'stony dull' note is elicited over a large pleural effusion. The area of dullness over the heart and liver is less extensive than would be expected from anatomical surface marking since aerated lung is interposed. A hyperresonant percussion note may be found over a lung or part of a lung which is markedly emphysematous and also over a large air-filled space, such as a pneumothorax. Below the diaphragm an underlying gas-containing viscus produces a tympanitic note.

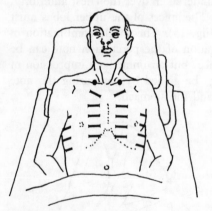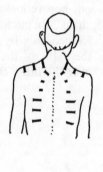

Fig. 15   Sites of percussion.

Auscultation

The patient should be asked to breathe in and out through the open mouth. The examiner should concentrate in turn on the following:

1. *breath sounds*—the character and intensity.
2. *added sounds*—nature, number and position in the respiratory cycle.
3. *vocal resonance*—the intensity and quality of the conducted voice.

To ensure that localised lesions are not overlooked, the stethoscope should be placed in many sites on the chest wall and the findings in equivalent positions on the two sides compared.

1. *Breath sounds* may be normal vesicular, diminished vesicular, vesicular with prolonged expiration, or bronchial.

Breath sounds are produced by vibrations of the vocal cords caused by the rapid flow of air through the larynx during inspiration and expiration. The sounds so produced are transmitted along the trachea and bronchi and through the lungs to the chest wall. In their passage through normal lungs the sounds are altered and, when heard through a stethoscope, they have a characteristic rustling quality to which the name *'vesicular'* is given. The intensity of these sounds increases steadily during inspiration and then quickly fades away during the first third of expiration.

Vesicular breath sounds are diminished in intensity if the chest wall is thick or if conduction of the sounds to the chest wall is reduced by shallow breathing, bronchial obstruction, emphysema, pneumothorax, pleural effusion or pleural thickening. The expiratory phase of vesicular breath sounds may be prolonged in the presence of airways obstruction, when it is often associated with expiratory rhonchi (p. 44).

Bronchial breath sounds are heard when sounds produced in the larynx are transmitted via patent airways to the chest wall through lung tissue which has lost its normal consistency thereby increasing sound conduction. Bronchial breath sounds are usually associated with pneumonic consolidation, but may also be present in other conditions such as pulmonary fibrosis or cavitation. The absence of bronchial breath sounds over an area of consolidation implies obstruction of the corresponding major bronchus. Since bronchial breath sounds indicate the presence of a pulmonary lesion, the criteria for their recognition must be unambiguous, namely:

(i) Both inspiratory and expiratory sounds must be loud and blowing in character, similar to those heard over the trachea.

(ii) The expiratory sound must be as long and as loud as the inspiratory sound.

(iii) There must be an audible pause between the end of the inspiratory sound and the beginning of the expiratory sound.

2. *Added sounds* heard on auscultation of the chest are of three types:

(i) Rhonchi (wheezes)
(ii) Crepitations (crackles)
(iii) Pleural rub (friction).

(i) *Rhonchi* are musical sounds of high, medium or low pitch produced by the passage of air through narrowed bronchi. In asthma, rhonchi are predominantly high and medium pitched and expiratory, while in bronchitis they are usually medium and low pitched and are audible during both inspiration and expiration.

(ii) *Crepitations* are non-musical sounds with a crackling quality. In some cases crepitations indicate excess secretions in the small airways. Such crepitations often increase in number temporarily after a short cough but may become less numerous or may disappear for a while after prolonged coughing. They are audible throughout inspiration.

In other cases crepitations are due to the explosive reopening, during inspiration, of peripheral airways which have been occluded during expiration by viscid exudate in the bronchioles or by thickening of the alveolar septa by oedema, inflammation or fibrosis. These crepitations are most numerous towards the end of inspiration and may be accompanied by rhonchi. They are not altered by coughing.

(iii) *A pleural* rub is a leathery or creaking sound produced by movement of the visceral over the parietal pleura when both surfaces have been roughened by a fibrinous exudate. It is usually audible at two separate stages of the respiratory cycle, towards the end of inspiration and just after the beginning of expiration. A pleural rub may be inaudible during quiet breathing, but becomes easily heard when the patient takes a deep breath. If there is difficulty in distinguishing between a low-pitched rhonchus and a pleural rub, auscultation should be repeated after a forceful cough. Rhonchi usually alter in character or disappear, while a rub remains unchanged. The temptation to elicit a rub should be resisted when severe pleural pain is present. In some cases a rub may be heard in the absence of pain, while in others severe pain may not be accompanied by a rub.

3. *Voice sounds* are transmitted from the larynx to the stethoscope on the chest wall and are modified in the same way as breath sounds; they normally have a muffled quality and are equal in intensity on the two sides. Vocal resonance is elicited by asking the patient to say 'one-one-one' (or 'ninety-nine') while the stethoscope is moved from one position to another, comparing the voice sounds in corresponding positions on the two sides. A localised reduction in breath sounds will be associated with decreased conduction of voice sounds, for example over a pleural effusion. Bronchial breath sounds are accompanied by increased conduction of spoken and whispered sounds.

Interpretation of physical signs

A summary of the principal physical signs found in consolidation, collapse, pleural effusion, pneumothorax and emphysema is given in Table 1.

Table 1 Summary of typical physical signs in some respiratory disorders

	Consolidation (as in lobar pneumonia)	Collapse (due to obstruction of major bronchus)	Pleural effusion (large)	Pneumothorax (large)	Emphysema (diffuse pulmonary)
Movement of chest wall	Reduced on side affected	Reduced on side affected	Reduced or absent on side affected	Reduced or absent on side affected	Symmetrically diminished
Mediastinal displacement	None	Towards side of lesion	Towards opposite side	Towards opposite side	None
Percussion Note	Dull	Dull	Stony dull	Hyperresonant	Normal or hypersonant over both lungs
Breath sounds	Bronchial	Diminished or absent	Diminished or absent	Diminished or absent	Diminished vesicular with prolonged expiration
Voice sounds	Increased	Reduced or absent	Reduced or absent	Reduced or absent	Normal or reduced
Added sounds	Crepitations	None	Pleural rub in some cases above effusion	None	None

4. The alimentary and the genito-urinary systems

THE HISTORY

1. The principal *symptoms of alimentary disease* are impaired appetite, difficulty in swallowing, heartburn, abdominal pain, nausea, vomiting, weight loss, gastrointestinal bleeding, alteration in bowel habit and jaundice. However many of these complaints may also be caused by disease in other systems; for example, epigastric pain may be due to myocardial infarction, vomiting may result from a cerebral tumour and jaundice may be due to haemolysis.

Anorexia (loss of appetite) can occur in many systemic diseases and also in some psychological disorders. There may also be local causes such as gastric carcinoma or hepatitis.

Dysphagia (difficulty in swallowing) should be regarded as a symptom demanding a physical explanation. It may comprise pain or a sensation of food sticking on swallowing or both.

Heartburn is a retrosternal burning discomfort occasionally experienced by many people. It occurs where there is an incompetent cardia and is common during pregnancy and with hiatus hernia.

Abdominal pain when analysed as described on page 3 almost invariably suggests the correct diagnosis. For example, duodenal ulceration causes pain which is usually localised to the epigastrium but may radiate to the back. It is boring in nature and of moderate severity. The pain usually lasts one half to two hours but can be relieved within 15 minutes by eating or by antacids. It often occurs before meals and may waken the patient at night. The pain tends to be episodic, occurring two or three times daily for several weeks but with remissions lasting from weeks to months.

Vomitus. Information of diagnostic value includes details about quantity, contents, colour and the patient's opinion about taste. For example, altered blood has the appearance of coffee grounds due to conversion of haemoglobin to acid haematin.

Bowels. Enquiry should be made as to the frequency, consistency and colour of the stool. Much altered blood causes a black stool (melaena). Any alteration in habit must be assessed as this may be an early symptom in malignant disease of the large bowel.

Jaundice associated with hepatitis or biliary obstruction causes dark urine and pale stools but haemolytic jaundice does not, because bilirubin is bound to albumin prior to its conjugation by the liver.

2. *Genito-urinary symptoms* depend on the site and nature of the lesion. However, many disorders of the kidneys do not cause local symptoms and they may present with the features of renal failure or hypertension. Pain may occur in the back between the 12th rib and iliac crest with radiation along the first lumbar dermatome as in renal colic from obstruction. A burning pain (*dysuria*) and frequency of micturition may be caused by inflammation of the bladder or urethra. The passage of blood (*haematuria*) may be the only manifestation of serious disease of the urinary tract. In the male, reduction in the force of the stream, hesitancy and terminal dribbling are suggestive of urethral obstruction from disease of the prostate gland. In the female, incontinence of urine on stress, e.g. from coughing, may follow stretching of the tissues of the pelvic floor at child birth.

Disorders of the female genital tract are commonly associated with vaginal discharge or a disturbance of the menstrual period but many other disease or psychological factors can also be responsible for menstrual changes. In the male, impotence often has a psychological basis; the physical causes include diabetic neuropathy.

THE PHYSICAL EXAMINATION

Examination of the mouth and throat are described on page 111.

Inspection and palpation constitute the main methods of examination of the abdomen with percussion and auscultation fulfilling supplementary functions. The patient should be examined in a good light and in warm surroundings; lying comfortably supine with the head on a pillow and the arms by the sides helps to relax the abdominal muscles. The skin

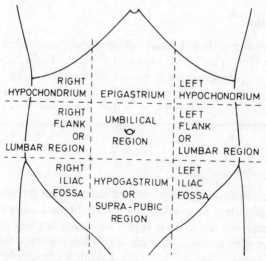

Fig. 16 Regions of the abdomen.

should be exposed from the xiphisternum to the pubis. The abdomen can be divided for descriptive purposes into nine regions by the intersection of two horizontal and two vertical planes (Fig. 16).

Inspection

The general shape and symmetry of the exposed abdomen is observed and attention paid to abnormalities of the skin and hair; enquiry should be made about scars if their cause is not already known; any abnormal veins, pulsations and other movements should also be noted. Pyloric obstruction can cause visible gastric peristalsis. The slow waves passing from the left subcostal area to and across the midline are most easily observed on tangential inspection. Small bowel peristalsis is seen as writhing movements in the central abdomen.

Palpation

The examiner should stand, sit or kneel comfortably beside the patient. The hands should be warm. Light, deep and bimanual palpation should be carried out. The patient should be asked to report if examination causes any discomfort and the patient's face should be watched for any indication of tenderness.

Light palpation

This should commence in an area remote from the site of any pain. Muscle tone is tested by gentle dipping movements as the hand is moved from region to region without breaking contact with the skin. Localised rigidity is usually associated with organic disease. Generalised rigidity commonly implies failure of the patient to relax but is also a feature of peritonitis when it is accompanied by tenderness. Inflammation of the peritoneum will produce *rebound pain* which is elicited by the sudden removal from the abdomen of the firmly applied hand.

Deep palpation

The abdomen should now be systematically palpated more deeply for organs and other masses using the whole palmar aspect of the fingers. In the normal abdomen it may be possible to feel such structures as a distended bladder, the aorta, faeces in the descending colon, the lower edge of the liver and lower pole of the right and occasionally of the left kidney (Fig. 17). The features of any mass should be noted as described on page 116 and also whether it descends on inspiration. The liver, gall bladder, spleen and kidneys move with respiration. Palpable enlargement of the gall bladder suggests either obstruction of the cystic duct, in which case the patient will not be jaundiced, or of the common bile duct when there is jaundice. Tenderness below the mid point of the right costal margin which is accentuated by, or limits, deep inspiration suggests acute cholecystitis (Murphy's sign).

Palpation during respiration

This method is used to feel for the liver, spleen and kidneys. A posterior hand, usually the left, should be lifted up between the 12th rib and the iliac crest, while the anterior hand, usually the right, should be placed over the organ to be palpated. The patient should be instructed to breathe deeply through the mouth, thereby pushing the organ or mass downwards into the waiting hands. When something is felt, the anterior hand should be moved to check on its characteristics.

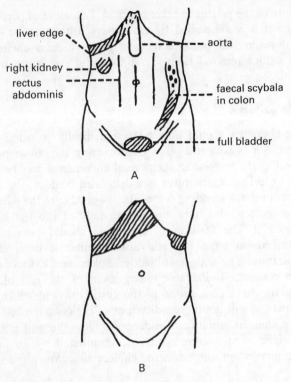

liver edge

right kidney

rectus
abdominis

aorta

faecal scybala
in colon

full bladder

A

B

Fig. 17 Abdominal palpation: A—normal findings;
B—hepatosplenomegaly.

1. Liver

The anterior hand should be placed flat, so that the sensing
fingers (index and middle) are lateral to the rectus muscle and
pointed upwards (Fig. 18A). The hand is pushed slightly
inwards and upwards until, at the height of inspiration, the
former pressure is released, allowing the finger to slip over
the edge of a palpable liver. It is then moved towards the
costal margin with each inspiration until the liver edge

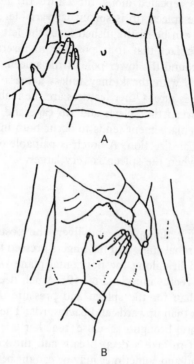

Fig. 18 Palpation of A—liver; B—spleen.

becomes palpable. The hand is then moved medially tracing the liver edge across the abdomen. Its shape, size, consistency and any tenderness are noted.

2. Spleen

The front hand is laid flat with the fingers at right angles to the left costal margin and pressed inwards and upwards (Fig. 18B). After each inspiration the anterior hand is moved upwards until the finger tips are under the costal margin and the process is repeated along the entire rib margin as the position of the spleen tip is somewhat variable.

The spleen can be distinguished from the left kidney most readily by the fact that it is possible to insert the fingers beneath and round the lower pole of the spleen. It is impossible to do this with the kidney unless a mass is projecting from it which is rare. Other features are the inability to place the hand between the spleen and rib cage and the fact that great splenic enlargement tends to occur both in a downward and in a medial direction. A notch is palpable on the medial border only when the spleen is very large.

3. Kidneys

As in palpating the spleen and liver, the posterior hand is placed in the renal angle and the fingers pressed forwards. The anterior hand lies along the horizontal plane with the finger tips over the rectus muscle (Fig. 19). Much deeper palpation is required than for the spleen and pressure directed backwards, rather than upwards and backwards. The fingers of the two hands are brought as close together as possible, the patient asked to take a deep breath and the kidney may be felt to descend and sometimes may be caught between the two hands. When the pressure is released, the kidney will slide upwards on expiration. Renal tenderness is usually greater posteriorly. The left kidney can be examined from the patient's right side (see Fig. 19C) but more effective palpation can be achieved from the patient's left (see Fig. 19B).

Percussion

The main value of abdominal percussion is to decide whether distension is due to gas, fluid (ascites) or a cystic or solid tumour. Percussion should be from resonant to dull with the

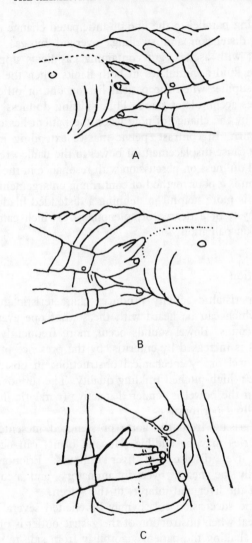

Fig. 19 Palpation of the kidneys: A & B—from the same side; C—from the opposite side.

finger lying parallel to the line of anticipated change of note. Gaseous distension and swellings overlaid by gas will be resonant; with ascites, gut containing gas floats uppermost while the fluid accumulates in both flanks when the patient is lying supine; when the patient lies on one or other side, the ascites accumulates there. This 'shifting dullness' can be detected by the change of note when the patient lies on each side in turn. In contrast, pelvic masses extending into the abdomen cause displacement of bowel to the flanks, resulting in central dullness on percussion with resonance in the flanks. Percussion is a poor method of confirming enlargement of the liver but is more helpful in defining a distended bladder, an ovarian cyst, or a degree of splenomegaly which cannot be detected on palpation.

Auscultation

Normal peristaltic activity produces characteristic gurgling sounds which can be heard with the stethoscope every five to ten seconds. Bowel sounds occur more frequently when peristalsis is increased by enteritis, by the presence of blood in the bowel or by mechanical obstruction; in obstruction they have a high-pitched tinkling quality. The sounds disappear when the bowel is rendered inactive (paralytic ileus) as in generalised peritonitis.

Bruits arising from the aorta or stenosed mesenteric or renal arteries may be audible. Hepatic bruits can occur in alcoholic liver disease and liver tumours. Friction may occasionally be heard over inflammatory and neoplastic disease of the liver and infarcts of the spleen.

A gastric succussion splash may be elicited several hours after a meal when obstruction of the gastric outlet is present, either by shaking the patient vigorously from side to side or by rapid dipping movements of the hand over the distended stomach.

Examination of the groins

The groins should be examined for enlarged lymph nodes; a few of about a centimetre in diameter are often palpable in healthy persons. The patient should be standing and should give a few good coughs for the detection of inguinal or femoral hernias. An impulse is present on coughing, but not if the hernia is strangulated. If a hernia is identified, an attempt may be made to reduce its contents by gentle sustained pressure.

Examination of male genitalia

The penis and scrotum are inspected and the testes, epididymes and vasa deferentia palpated gently. Examination of a scrotal swelling should follow the principles laid down on page 116. It is necessary to ascertain that the swelling originates in the scrotum and is not an inguinal hernia. A hydrocele can usually be transilluminated (p. 118) and can be

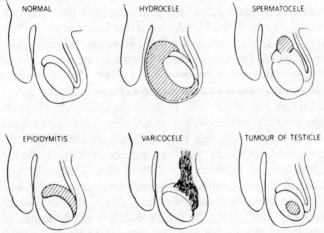

Fig. 20   Swellings of the scrotum.

differentiated from a spermatocele and a cyst of the epididymis by its relationship to the testis as illustrated in Figure 20. The possibility that a hydrocele may obscure a testicular tumour must not be overlooked and in each case the testis must be palpated with care.

Digital examination of the rectum

Many errors in diagnosis have been made because examination of the rectum has been omitted. The patient, chaperoned if necessary, should be informed of the need to examine the back passage. If the examiner is right-handed, the patient should lie curled up in the left lateral position with a maximal degree of flexion consistent with comfort. The buttocks should be at the edge of a couch or bed. The examiner's right forefinger, protected by a fingerstall or glove, should be smeared with a lubricant. Using a good light, the perianal skin should be examined, particularly for thrombosed external haemorrhoids or fistulae. The forefinger tip is placed on the anal margin and with steady pressure on the sphincter the finger is inserted gently through the anal canal into the rectum (Fig. 21A & B). If the examination is very painful, an anal fissure is likely to be present and the examination should be discontinued. The exploring finger should feel round the whole extent of the rectum; this is normally empty and the walls smooth and soft. Posteriorly, the coccyx and sacrum can be felt through the rectal wall while anteriorly in the male the prostate is readily felt (Fig. 21C). The normal gland is smooth and has a fairly firm consistency with the contours of miniature buttocks represented by a shallow median groove between the lateral lobes. Haemorrhoids which are not thrombosed and normal seminal vesicles cannot be felt. In the female the firm round cervix uteri can be felt anteriorly (Fig. 21D); the presence of a vaginal tampon or pessary may also be felt and can confuse the novice.

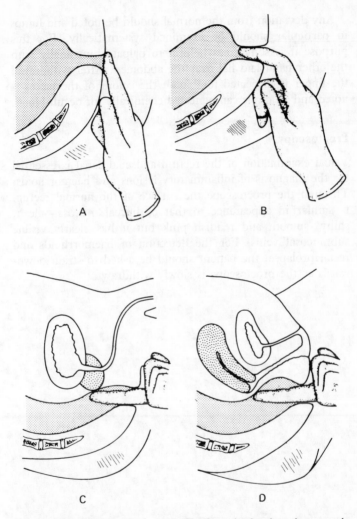

Fig. 21 Examination of the rectum. The finger is placed on the external sphincter (A) and inserted into the rectum (B). The hand is then rotated and the most prominent features are the prostate in the male (C) and the cervix in the female (D).

Any deviation from the normal should be noted and lumps in particular should be examined systematically. For this purpose it is sometimes helpful to palpate bimanually with the other hand laid flat over the abdomen. After withdrawal the finger is inspected for blood; the colour of the faeces is noted and a sample can be tested chemically for occult blood.

Proctoscopy

Visual examination of the rectum and anal canal is essential for the diagnosis of inflammatory lesions and haemorrhoids. Through the proctoscope the surface of the normal rectum is similar in appearance to that of buccal mucosa—clean, shiny, smooth and reddish pink but it has clearly visible submucosal veins. For the detection of haemorrhoids and rectal prolapse, the patient should be asked to strain downwards as the proctoscope is slowly withdrawn.

5. The nervous system

THE HISTORY

The object of taking a neurological history is to graph the course of symptoms in terms of their severity and time relationships. In this way the pattern of past and current symptoms can be interpreted within a framework of recognised stereotypes of neurological disorders. After listening to the patient's account of the illness, specific questions should be asked about the principal neurological symptoms described below. It is essential, as in other systems, to make every effort to obtain the precise meaning of the patient's complaint. For example, a decision should be made as to whether the terms 'giddiness' or 'dizziness' refer to a disorder of balance with some sense of rotation (*vertigo*) or to the wobbly, vague feelings that precede a faint or are associated with anxiety.

Headache should be analysed as for any other pain (p. 3). Headache is often caused by nervous tension but when due to an expanding intracranial lesion it may be associated with vomiting, focal symptoms or impairment of consciousness.

Unconsciousness may be of sudden onset; every endeavour should be made to obtain an eye witness account. For example, the description can be diagnostic of an epileptic fit.

Visual difficulties include photophobia (intolerance of light), diplopia (double vision), and impairment of vision. Episodes

61

of diplopia and blurred vision (amblyopia) are frequent in multiple sclerosis. A transient visual disorder is a common prelude to a migrainous headache.

Deafness is common in the elderly and minor degrees are often overlooked. It may be associated with buzzing or ringing in the ears (*tinnitus*).

Paraesthesiae (tingling or numbness) are due to involvement of sensory pathways between the peripheral nerve endings up to, and including, the parietal cortex. Localised *weakness* is due to a disorder of the upper or lower motor neurone, myoneural junction or muscle.

Sphincter disturbances most frequently involve bladder function. Sensory loss leads to retention with overflow. Motor loss usually causes urgency yet the patient cannot pass urine at will. Combined sensory and motor loss causes an automatic bladder which sometimes can be emptied at will by manual pressure on the lower abdomen. Occasionally in such cases the bladder is spastic and incontinence is persistent.

THE PHYSICAL EXAMINATION

The detailed examination of specific nerve functions should be preceded by an assessment of the patient's intellectual abilities (p. 7), gait (p. 99) and speech.

Once the general assessment has been completed, the motor system, the sensory system, the reflexes and the cranial nerves should be examined.

Speech

Impairment of language function (*dysphasia*) may be *expressive* (*motor*), when patients understand what is said and know what they wish to say but are unable to say it. It is *receptive* (*sensory*) when there is impairment of comprehension; this is tested by asking the patient to carry out commands of gradually increasing difficulty, for example, 'Close your eyes', 'Raise your right arm and then bow your head.' The responses will often reveal a combination of receptive and expressive defects called *global dysphasia*.

Speech may be normal in its use of language but impaired because of difficulty in articulation (*dysarthria*) due to defective movements of lips, tongue or palate, or to a combination thereof. Dysarthria may be caused by diseases of the cerebellum or its connections when the speech becomes scanning or staccato, or by disease involving the motor neurones when the words become slurred and indistinct. Abnormalities of speech may also arise from impairment of sound production (dysphonia) usually due to lesions of the vocal cord but sometimes resulting from disorders of the neuro-muscular supply or to inadequate expiratory air flow.

THE EXAMINATION OF THE MOTOR SYSTEM

The motor pathways are shown in Figure 22. Assessment of motor function involves inspection of muscle bulk and testing of tone, power, coordination and fine movements. The scheme for examination of the nervous system is usually applied first to the upper limbs and then repeated for the lower limbs, though some prefer to examine the patients from the feet upwards. A useful preliminary manoeuvre requires the patient to hold the arms outstretched with fingers spread, first with eyes open and then closed. Failure to maintain the position suggests a neurological disorder.

Inspection

Muscle wasting

The examiner should inspect the shape and bulk of the patient's musculature; asymmetry is more suggestive of an abnormality than is symmetrical wasting.

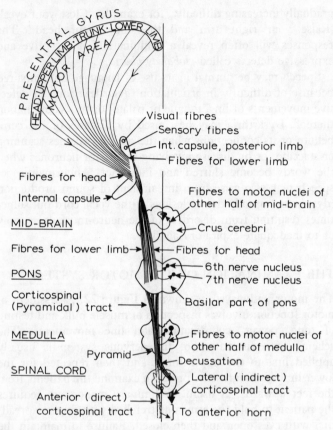

Fig. 22 The motor pathways.

Fasciculation

This is due to the spontaneous contraction of large groups of muscle fibres or of whole motor units. Fasciculations are visible twitches occurring sporadically in different parts of the muscle and suggest a lesion in the proximal part of the lower motor neurone.

Involuntary movements

Tremors result from alternate contraction and relaxation of groups of muscles producing rhythmic oscillations about a joint or group of joints. The rate and amplitude of any tremor should be estimated. The commonest is the exaggeration of the 10 per second physiological tremor which underlies all apparently smooth movements. This can be demonstrated by laying a sheet of paper over the outstretched fingers. An increase in physiological tremor is often found in anxious patients, in hyperthyroidism and in alcoholics. A slower, 4 per second, coarse tremor is a feature of parkinsonism and commonly involves adduction-abduction movements of the thumb with flexion and extension movements of the fingers. It is halted by purposive movement.

Choreiform movements are irregular, jerky, ill-sustained and appear semi-purposive. They affect different muscles unpredictably in quick succession. This distinguishes choreiform movements from the similar but much commoner *habit spasm* or *tic*, which is a repetitive and stereotyped movement.

Athetoid movements are slow and writhing and principally affect the distal parts of the limbs.

Various extrapyramidal disorders lead to parkinsonian, choreiform and athetoid movements.

Tone

Tone may be defined clinically as the resistance felt when a joint is moved passively. During its assessment the patient must be relaxed and neither resist nor assist the movements. Co-operation is best achieved with the patient lying comfortably in a supine position. It may help to ask the patient to relax or to 'go floppy'. The elbow, wrist, knee and hip joints should be put through the full range of movement, manipulating each joint rapidly to start with and then more slowly. A useful assessment of tone can be made at the wrist by

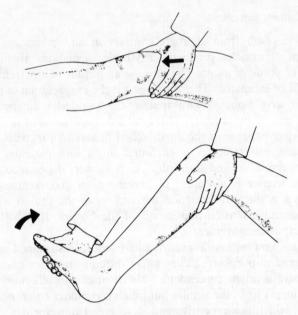

Fig. 23 Testing for knee and ankle clonus.

shaking the forearm and at the ankle by rocking the leg to and fro on the bed. Tone may be increased (hypertonia) or decreased (hypotonia).

Hypertonia is of two distinct types, spasticity and rigidity. Spasticity is characteristic of upper motor neurone lesions and produces an increasing resistance to the first few degrees of passive movement then as the movement continues there is a sudden lessening of resistance ('clasp knife' spasticity). Rigidity is characteristic of disorders of the basal ganglia and produces a sustained resistance throughout the range of movement ('lead-pipe' rigidity). The 'cogwheel' rigidity of parkinsonism is the jerky resistance to passive movement which occurs when tremor is super-imposed on rigidity.

Hypotonia or decreased resistance is more difficult to assess unless the lesion is unilateral when comparison can be made with the normal side. Hypotonia occurs in lower motor neurone or cerebellar lesions, and often during the first few days following sudden upper motor neurone damage.

Clonus is the rhythmic repetition of involuntary muscular contractions evoked by a sudden passive stretch of a muscle. A few beats of clonus elicited in anxious patients may not be significant. Sustained clonus (i.e. contractions which continue as long as stretch is applied) is indicative of a lesion of the upper motor neurone. Patellar clonus is elicited by sharply pushing the patella towards the foot whilst the patient lies supine and relaxed with the knee extended. Ankle clonus is produced by a brisk dorsiflexion of the foot (Fig. 22).

Power

Power can be tested by asking the patient to move a joint and then maintain its position whilst the examiner forcefully over-comes it. This is called *isometric testing*. Alternatively the patient may be asked to put a joint through a full range of movement using maximal power while the examiner opposes the movement. This is *isotonic testing*. Both methods are effec-tive but the latter is more sensitive in detecting minor degrees of weakness. Power should be assessed both proximally and distally and as each movement is examined it should be immediately compared with that in the other limb. Occasionally all muscle groups will require to be assessed; usually it is only necessary to test selectively.

Coordination

The smooth and accurate performance of purposeful move-ments requires intact motor, sensory and cerebellar functions. Any lesion which causes weakness may be accompanied by clumsiness but incoordination is particularly prominent in sensory and cerebellar ataxia. *Sensory ataxia* results from defective proprioception and can to some extent be mitigated by visual feedback i.e. it is worse when the eyes are closed (p. 73) *Cerebellar ataxia* is not susceptible to visual compensation.

Rapid, alternating movements are rendered irregular in force and rhythm by cerebellar disorders *dysdiadokokinesis*. They may be tested by rapid pronation and supination of the forearm e.g. quickly slapping the examiner's palm with the front and back of the hand alternately. Patients vary widely in their abilities to carry out such movements. Most perform the tests more precisely and rapidly with the dominant hand and are somewhat clumsy when using the other hand.

Coordination of the upper limbs is assessed by the finger–nose test (Fig. 24A). The patient is asked to hold the arm outstretched and then to touch the tip of the nose with the tip of the index finger. The patient with sensory ataxia performs these acts better when the eyes are open. If cerebellar ataxia is present, the patient may overshoot the target even when the eyes are open (dysmetria) and movements are clumsy and jerky especially as the nose is approached ('intention tremor').

Coordination of the lower limbs is assessed by the examination of the gait (p. 99) and the heel-knee test; the patient places one heel on the opposite knee and then slides the heel down the front of the shin to the ankle and back again (Fig. 24B).

Assessment of fine movements

The ability to carry out small, precise, coordinated finger movements can be assessed by asking the patient to make 'piano-playing' individual finger movements as rapidly as possible with each hand in turn. These are often impaired at an early stage in lesions of the upper motor neurones or the extrapyramidal system. In addition, the patient should be

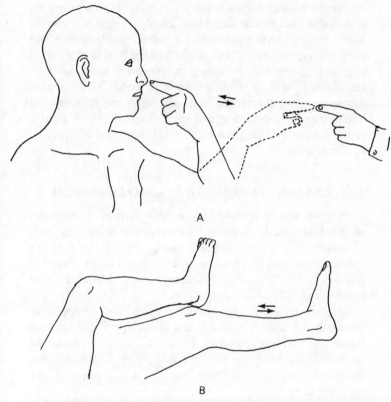

Fig. 24 Tests of limb coordination: A—finger-nose test; B—heel-shin test.

observed carrying out common, everyday activities which
demand precise coordination of finger movements, such as
fastening buttons or tying knots.

Testing for dyspraxia

Difficulty in the performance of more complex movements
may be observed in the absence of incoordination, weakness
or sensory defect. This suggests an inability to formulate and

synthesise movement patterns (dyspraxia). If this suspicion is aroused, the patient should be asked to carry out specific tasks, such as dressing, winding a watch, combing hair and putting on spectacles. These simple tests of the parietal cortex may be supplemented by asking the patient to draw geometrical figures such as a square or a triangle. Patients with dyspraxia write slowly and with difficulty; the formation of letters may be incomplete and their size variable. A sample of the patient's writing can be a useful record for comparison at a later date.

THE EXAMINATION OF THE SENSORY SYSTEM

Testing for sensation should involve comparison of both sides of the body. It is important to develop efficient methods of examination since repetition causes loss of the patient's concentration and cooperation. Interpretation of the abnormal findings in the light of neuroanatomy leads to localisation of lesions (Figs 25, 26).

Bilateral selective impairment of pain and temperature sensation indicates a central lesion of the spinal cord, as the fibres relay in the posterior horns and cross to form the spinothalamic tract on the opposite side. It follows that unilateral selective impairment indicates a tract lesion on the opposite side.

Selective impairment of position and vibration sense indicates damage to the nerve fibres which ascend in the ipsilateral posterior columns or rarely to a lesion of their central connections on the opposite side above the medulla.

Touch

The patient should be asked, with the eyes closed, to report the touch of a point of cotton wool which should be applied at irregular time intervals, comparing one side with the other,

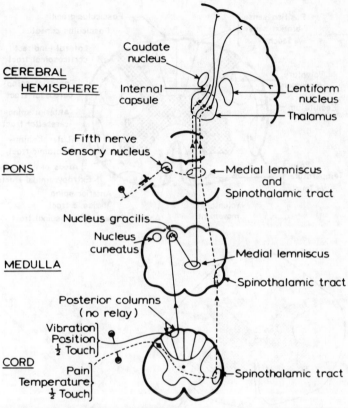

Fig. 25 The main sensory pathways.

and mapping out in detail, areas of altered sensation on limbs or trunk. This is best undertaken by testing from abnormal to normal.

Pain

The patient should be asked, with the eyes closed, to distinguish between stimulation with the point and the head

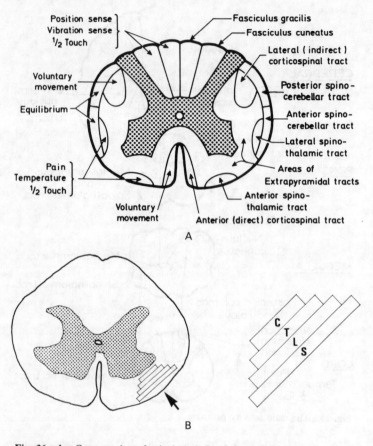

Fig. 26 A—Cross section of spinal cord. B—Spinothalamic tracts: cervical segments (C) lie centrally with the thoracic (T), lumbar (L) and sacral segments (S) lying progressively more laterally.

of a pin. It is important to ensure that each dermatome is tested with the sharp stimulus. Pain sensation should be contrasted between opposite sides of the body. Any area of impaired sensation should be mapped out.

Temperature sensation

This is tested only occasionally in confirmation of the findings on pinprick. The patient, with the eyes closed, attempts to distinguish between tubes containing either hot or cold water applied in random sequence to the skin.

Joint position sense

Loss of joint position sense may be suggested from the history, for example if the patient complains of difficulty in walking in the dark. This may be tested by asking the patient to stand upright with feet together. Loss of balance on closing the eyes suggests sensory ataxia (Rombergism), and with the eyes open, suggests cerebellar ataxia.

The position sense at individual joints is tested by passive movements. The distal parts of the limbs are usually affected initially and therefore movements of the interphalangeal joint of the index finger and great toe should be tested first. With

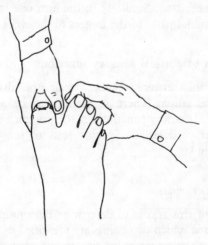

Fig. 27 Testing joint position sense in the great toe.

the thumb and forefinger of the right hand the examiner grips the terminal phalanx while the more proximal phalanx is held by the other hand. The distal phalanx is then extended or flexed. When it is clear that the test is understood, the patient is asked to close the eyes and to indicate the direction of movement, care being taken to ensure that the examiner's finger does not rub against the patient's other digits (Fig. 27). The normal minimal range of movement which can be appreciated should be learned by practice. Only if joint position sense is impaired peripherally need similar tests be employed at more proximal joints.

Vibration sense

The patient is asked to describe the sensation produced by a vibrating tuning fork, ideally with a frequency of 128 cycles/sec, placed on the dorsum of the big toe. Where vibration sense is lost, the tuning fork should be moved proximally in order to establish the level at which it is normally appreciated. Similarly in the arm one may proceed from the terminal parts of the fingers to the wrist and elbow.

Examination of cortical sensory functions

Lesions of the sensory cortex impair the discriminative aspects of sensation. There is nothing to be achieved by testing cortical sensory functions in the presence of a peripheral nerve or cord lesion. Specific tests of sensory cortical function include:

Two-point discrimination

The object of this test is to determine the minimal distance of separation at which two points are identified as two distinct stimuli. Over the finger pulps two points separated by only

2 to 3 mm are normally so recognised. Over the leg the distance may exceed 50 mm. One or both points of a pair of dividers, which can be specially calibrated to show the amount of separation of their points, should be applied randomly over the skin of the fingers. The patient, with the eyes closed, is asked to say if one or two points can be felt after each stimulation. An opened-out paper clip makes a readily available 'instrument'.

Stereognosis

The patient, with eyes closed, is asked to identify objects by palpation. Articles such as a key, coin, pen or a wallet are suitable. An alternative method, also suitable for the lower limbs, is to ask the patient to identify unseen numbers outlined on the skin.

Sensory inattention

This tests perception of simultaneous stimuli at corresponding sites on both sides of the body. It is first essential to demonstrate that a stimulus, either touch or pinprick, is felt when separately applied to an appropriate point on each side. If bilateral stimuli are delivered simultaneously, that on one side only may be perceived when there is a lesion in the sensory cortex. The test should be repeated several times, the patient's eyes being closed throughout, in order to confirm that the inattention is consistent.

THE EXAMINATION OF REFLEXES

The reflex arc consists of an afferent pathway triggered by stimulating a receptor, an efferent system which activates an effector organ and a communication between these two components. Since a reflex response to an appropriate stimulus is involuntary, disturbances of reflexes afford objective signs of neural dysfunction and any interruption of the arc will result in loss or diminution of the reflex. Routine physical examination should include common tendon and cutaneous reflexes.

Tendon reflexes

Biceps, triceps, supinator, knee and ankle reflexes (jerks) are evoked by a brisk stretch of the appropriate tendon; this is most efficiently done by a tap from a tendon hammer. The tendon, not the muscles should be struck as mechanical stimulation of a muscle belly produces a contraction which is independent of the reflex arc. The patient should be in a comfortable, relaxed position which allows the examiner easy access to the limbs. Convenient positions and methods are illustrated in Figure 28. A normal tendon reflex results in a sudden variable degree of muscle contraction which then rapidly returns to normal. The response on the two sides should be compared. Tendon reflexes may be increased, decreased, absent or delayed.

Increased tendon reflexes

Abnormal increase in the response to tendon stretch results from upper motor neurone lesions. Reflexes may be brisker than usual as a result of anxiety and a decision as to whether a reflex is abnormally brisk may depend upon other evidence such as the plantar response (see below). Hyperreflexia in the upper limbs can be confirmed by Hoffmann's test. This involves suddenly releasing the flexed distal interphalangeal joint of the patient's middle finger. When positive the thumb and forefinger quickly flex in response.

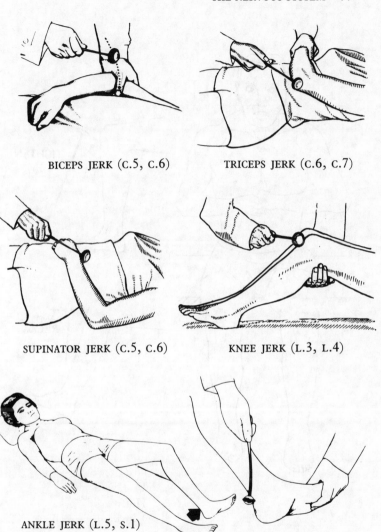

BICEPS JERK (C.5, C.6)

TRICEPS JERK (C.6, C.7)

SUPINATOR JERK (C.5, C.6)

KNEE JERK (L.3, L.4)

ANKLE JERK (L.5, S.1)

Fig. 28 Eliciting tendon reflexes (principal segmental innervations).

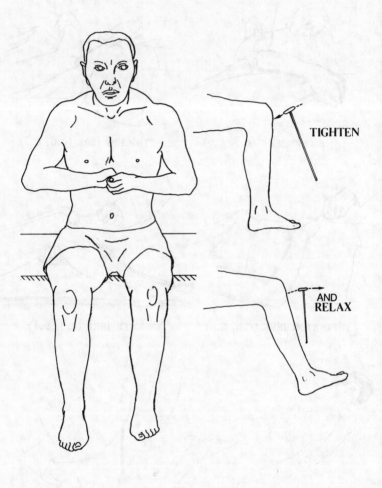

Fig. 29 Reinforcing the knee jerk.

Decreased, absent or delayed tendon reflexes

The significance of depressed tendon reflexes requires careful appraisal because they are difficult or even impossible to elicit in a few normal people. Usually, however, absence of one or more tendon jerks denotes a neural lesion. When no response is obtained, the absence of the reflex should be confirmed by 'reinforcement'. To reinforce the knee and ankle jerks the patient may be asked to hook the fingers together and then forcibly to attempt to pull one hand away from the other without disengaging the fingers (Fig. 29). Reinforcement of the reflexes in the upper limbs may best be obtained by

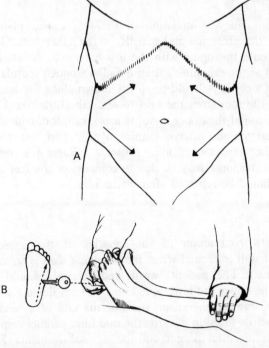

Fig. 30 Sites to elicit A—the abdominal reflexes; B—the plantar response.

asking the patient to clench the jaws or to push the knees hard together. A further attempt is immediately made to elicit the tendon jerk and then the patient is instructed to relax.

Delayed muscle relaxation, particularly noticeable in the ankle jerk, is characteristic of hypothyroidism.

Superficial reflexes

These consist of muscular contractions evoked by cutaneous stimulation. The plantar response is the best known and most important.

Plantar reflex

Except in infancy, stimulation of the sole causes plantar flexion of the great toe and usually of the other toes. The patient should lie supine with the legs extended. A blunted point such as the examiner's thumb nail, a wooden spatula or the end of a car key should be slowly drawn along the lateral border of the foot from the heel towards the little toe (Fig. 30B). A lesion of the upper motor neurone causes dorsiflexion of the great toe and often a fanning of the other four toes; this is the extensor plantar response (*Babinski's sign*). Absence of response may be due to coldness of the feet and the test should be repeated after warming.

Abdominal reflexes

Normally a contraction of the muscles of the anterior abdominal wall is evoked when the overlying skin is stroked or scratched. The patient, warm and relaxed, should lie supine. The upper and lower quadrants on each side are stimulated by drawing an orange stick or the end of a tendon hammer across the skin towards the mid line, parallel respectively with the costal margins and the inguinal ligaments (Fig. 30). The reflexes may be absent if the abdominal wall is lax.

Absent responses in a young patient strongly suggest an upper motor neurone lesion for which there is usually corroborative evidence.

THE EXAMINATION OF THE CRANIAL NERVES

The olfactory (first cranial) nerve

Loss of sense of smell (*anosmia*) is much more commonly due to nasal disease than to neurological causes and hence enquiry should be made about nasal catarrh and the patency of the nasal passageways tested by asking the patient to sniff as each nostril is occluded in turn by finger pressure. The olfactory nerve is not usually tested unless the possibility of a neurological lesion which could cause anosmia is suspected, for example a tumour of the anterior cerebral fossa. Then the patient, with eyes closed, is asked to identify common odours such as an orange or tobacco but avoiding pungent substances such as ammonia; each nostril is tested separately, the other being occluded by finger pressure.

The optic (second cranial) nerve

The optic nerve head and fundus should be examined by ophthalmoscopy as described on page 121.

Visual acuity

The acuity of distant vision is measured by the ability of the patient, with each eye in turn, to read standard *Snellen types* at a distance of six metres. The results are recorded as 6/6, 6/18, etc., the latter meaning that at 6 m the patient can just read what should be readable at 18 m. Near vision can be tested by using standard reading charts such as the *Jaeger card*; the smallest print which can be read by each eye should be recorded. Spectacles should be worn if required.

Visual fields

Defects in the visual fields resulting from lesions of the visual pathways are shown in Figure 31. The visual fields are assessed clinically by the technique of confrontation. A white-headed pin or a waggling forefinger are handy test objects. The patient covers one eye and looks at the opposing eye of

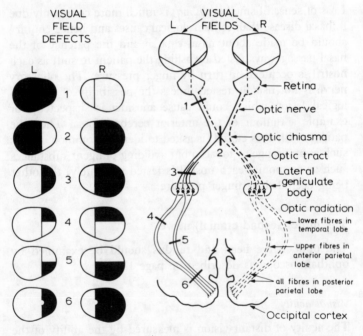

Fig. 31 Visual field defects: 1. Total loss of vision in one eye due to a lesion of the optic nerve. 2. Bitemporal hemianopia due to compression of the optic chiasma. 3. Right homonymous hemianopia from a lesion of the optic tract. 4. Upper right quadrantic hemianopia from a lesion of the lower fibres of the optic radiation in the temporal lobe. 5. Less commonly a lower quadrantic hemianopia occurs from a lesion of the upper fibres of the optic radiation in the anterior part of the parietal lobe. 6. Right homonymous hemianopia with sparing of the macula from a lesion of the optic radiation in the posterior part of the parietal lobe.

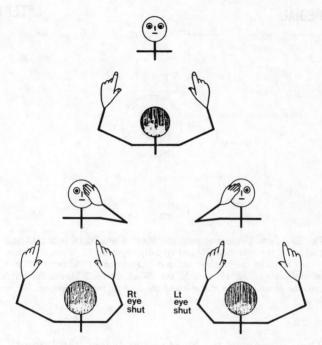

Fig. 32 Testing the visual fields.

the examiner (Fig. 32). The test is invalidated if the patient looks away. The clinician examines the outer limits by bringing the target into the field of vision from the periphery at several points on the circumference. The direction of approach should be radial and distributed over upper and lower quadrants of nasal and temporal aspects of the visual fields. Central field defects may also be mapped by moving the test object within the limits of the field. After each eye is examined separately the clinician checks for visual inattention by asking the patient to report if the test object is moved on one or both sides simultaneously (see Fig. 32).

MEDIAL   **LATERAL**

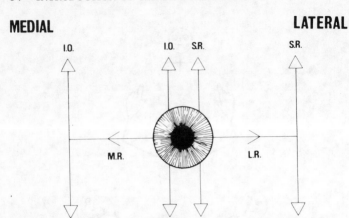

Fig. 33 Testing ocular movements. Medical and lateral recti (MR and LR) move the eyes medially and laterally respectively. When the eye is turned medially the superior oblique (SO) depresses the eye and the inferior oblique (IO) elevates the eye. When the eye is turned laterally, the superior rectus elevates the eye and the inferior rectus depresses the eye.

The oculomotor, trochlear and abducent (third, fourth and sixth cranial) nerves

The sixth cranial nerve supplies the lateral rectus muscle which moves the eye laterally. The fourth nerve supplies the superior oblique muscle which is a pure depressor when the eye is adducted. All the other eye movements, raising the upper lid and constriction of the pupil are controlled by the third nerve (Fig. 33). The superior tarsal muscle, supplied by the sympathetic, also raises the upper lid slightly (see Horner's syndrome p. 111).

Inspection of eyes

Any asymmetry should be noted, such as drooping of an

eyelid (ptosis) or difference in the widths of the palpebral fissures.

The pupils are normally round, regular in outline and equal. Their size varies with the intensity of ambient lighting but is usually between 3 and 5 mm in diameter. Constriction of the pupil is less than 3 mm is known as *miosis* while dilatation above 5 mm in average illumination is called *mydriasis*.

Pupillary reflexes

If a light is shone into one eye, both pupils constrict. The

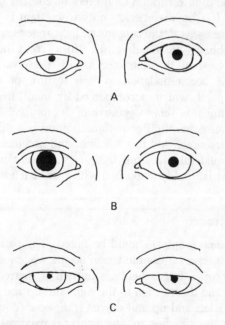

Fig. 34 Pupillary abnormalities: A—Right Horner's syndrome (ptosis and miosis); B—Right Holmes-Adie pupil; C—Argyll Robertson pupils with bilateral ptosis.

reaction of the pupil on the side stimulated is the *direct light reflex* and the constriction of the other pupil is the *consensual light reflex*. The speed and extent of constriction should be assessed in each eye separately, shielding the other from the light while doing so in order to test both direct and consensual reflexes. The light should approach from the side in order to avoid an accommodation response. The *reaction of accommodation* refers to the constriction of the pupils which occurs when the eyes converge on a near object. The patient is first asked to gaze into the distance and then to look at a finger placed near the patient's nose.

Impairment or absence of the pupillary reaction to light may be due to interruption of afferent or efferent sides of the reflex arc. If a pupil constricts only when light is shone into the opposite eye (i.e. the consensual light reflex is preserved), the eye is blind, but the efferent pathway from the midbrain is intact. Lost of the light reflex with preservation of the reaction of accommodation is one feature of the *Argyll Robertson pupil*, which, accompanied by small, irregular and unequal pupils, is very suggestive of neurosyphilis (Fig. 34). The Holmes-Adie pupil or myotonic pupil is a dilated pupil which reacts sluggishly to both light and accommodation. It is often unilateral, does not indicate significant neurological disease and is usually associated with loss of tendon reflexes.

Ocular movements

Any *strabismus* (squint) should be noted. The patient should be asked to report if double vision occurs while following the movement of a finger held about half a metre away and moved up and down, then to the right and up and down, and then to the left and up and down. If *diplopia* (double vision) is present, the direction in which there is maximal separation of the images should be ascertained. The peripheral image is the false one and attributable to the eye whose movement is impaired.

Disordered movements may result from lesions of (1) ocular muscles (myopathies), (2) neuromuscular junctions (myasthenia gravis), (3) ocular nerves or their nuclei, (4) internuclear and supranuclear connections.

Nystagmus

The presence of vertical, horizontal or rotatory nystagmus, i.e., involuntary rhythmic oscillations of the eyes, should be sought during the testing of ocular movements. The direction of gaze in which nystagmus occurs should be noted. Nystagmus is described as 'pendular' when the oscillations about a central point are equal in rate and amplitude. Pendular nystagmus may occur in any plane and most commonly results from a defect in macular vision. Jerking nystagmus is composed of quick and slow oscillations about a central point.

The quicker phase is arbitrarily used to define the direction of nystagmus. Thus 'nystagmus to the right' does not refer to the direction of gaze in which nystagmus occurs but to the direction of the quick phase. Jerking nystagmus indicates a disturbance in the vestibular apparatus, the eighth cranial nerve or its connections with the brain stem and cerebellum. Peripheral lesions affecting the vestibular apparatus or nerve produce a uni-directional nystagmus irrespective of the direction of gaze. In contrast, central lesions in the brain stem or cerebellum produce bidirectional nystagmus (the direction changing with the direction of gaze). Lesions of the medial longitudinal bundle produce bidirectional nystagmus more marked in the abducting eye (dysconjugate or ataxic nystagmus).

The trigeminal (fifth cranial) nerve

Sensory function

Light touch and pain sensations are tested in the territory of the three sensory divisions using cotton wool and pin prick respectively (Fig. 35A) and comparing the two sides of the forehead, the cheeks and the jaw by the methods described for sensory testing in general (p. 70).

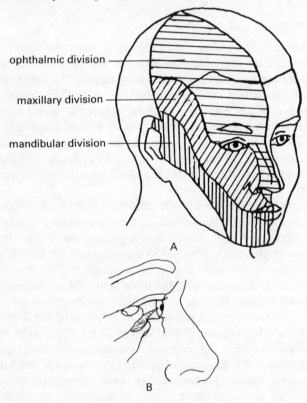

ophthalmic division

maxillary division

mandibular division

Fig. 35 A—divisions of the trigeminal nerve; B—eliciting the corneal reflex.

Motor function

The muscles of mastication are tested by asking the patient to open the jaw against resistance; it will deviate towards the side of any unilateral weakness of the pterygoid muscles. Also, as the teeth are clenched, the masseter muscles should be palpated and an estimate made of their bulk and symmetry.

Reflexes

The *corneal reflex* comprises a brisk closure of the eye evoked by touching the cornea gently with a wisp of cotton wool. The wisp must be introduced from the side so that the patient does not see it approaching (Fig. 35B). The afferent part of the reflex arc is the first division of the trigeminal nerve; the motor limb is the facial nerve.

The *jaw jerk* is analogous to the tendon reflexes in the

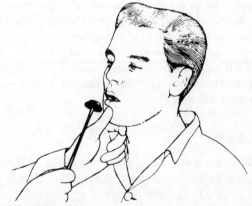

Fig. 36 Eliciting the jaw jerk.

limbs. The patient is asked to let the mouth hang open. The examiner places a thumb on the chin and then strikes the thumb downwards with a tendon hammer (Fig. 36). The afferent and efferent pathways are provided by the fifth cranial nerve. A pathologically brisk jaw jerk denotes a bilateral upper motor neurone lesion.

The facial (seventh cranial) nerve

Motor function

Signs of facial paralysis may be obvious on inspection with absence of wrinkling of the forehead, drooping of the corner of the mouth or flattening of the nasolabial fold. Movements of the upper part of the face should be compared with activity in the lower face; the patient should be asked to frown, wrinkle the forehead and close the eyes as tightly as possible, show the teeth and blow out the cheeks or whistle.

Impaired facial movements may be due to disturbance of supranuclear motor pathways, to affections of the seventh cranial nerve itself or, more rarely, to myasthenia gravis or a myopathy. Because upper facial movements are innervated from both sides of the cortex, unilateral upper motor neurone lesions characteristically weaken movements of the lower part of the face more than those of the upper face, whereas a lower motor neurone lesion affects both equally. Involuntary movements such as blinking or those due to smiling and other emotional expressions may be preserved in a lesion of the upper motor neurone.

Sensory function

Taste sensation from the anterior two-thirds of the tongue is transmitted by the facial nerve through the chorda tympani. It is not assessed routinely but when appropriate, the primary tastes, sweet, salt, bitter and sour, should be tested using sugar or saccharine, salt, quinine and vinegar respectively. The tongue should be protruded while the examiner holds it gently in a swab. The test substances are placed on each side in turn and the patient is asked to identify the tastes by pointing to the word 'sweet', 'salt', 'bitter', or 'sour', on a card.

The vestibulocochlear (eight cranial) nerve

The eighth cranial nerve comprises two distinct components, vestibular and auditory. Vestibular functions cannot effectively be evaluated at the bedside.

Hearing should be tested in each ear in turn by whispering close to the patient's ear with the opposite ear occluded by finger pressure over the meatus. Further information about the type of deafness can be obtained by using a tuning fork giving 256 cycles/second (though 128 c/sec will serve). Its base is placed on the mastoid bone until the sound fades; the sound should still be audible when the tip is held over the meatus (*Rinne's test*). With a conduction defect due to wax or a foreign body in the meatus or disease of the middle ear, bone may be better than air conduction. In auditory nerve damage (perceptive deafness) the normal relationship is preserved. If hearing is impaired or if earache is a problem, the external ear passages and the drums should be inspected through an auriscope (page 112).

The glossopharyngeal (ninth cranial) nerve

Many of the functions of the glossopharyngeal nerve are intermingled with those of the tenth cranial nerve.

The sensory supply to the posterior third of the tongue and the pharynx can be tested by touching these areas with the point of an orange stick. The procedure is unpleasant and should be performed only when it is important to define ninth nerve function precisely. Touching the posterior wall of the pharynx evokes the 'gag' reflex whose afferent and efferent paths are the glossopharyngeal and vagus nerves respectively.

The vagus (tenth cranial) nerve

Lesions of the vagus nerve or its recurrent laryngeal branch may give rise to dysphonia (p. 63); interruption of its motor fibres high in the neck will give a nasal quality to the voice by impairing the movement of the palate.

The soft palate should be inspected and its movements observed as the patient utters a prolonged 'ah'. In bilateral palsies the palate will not elevate; in unilateral lesions one side of the palate does not rise, and the uvula moves towards the normal side. Movement of the posterior pharyngeal wall should be observed during phonation. If one side is paralysed, it tends to move laterally towards the normal side.

The spinal accessory (eleventh cranial) nerve

This nerve is tested by examining the bulk and power of the sternomastoid and trapezius muscles. When testing the sternomastoids it is useful to examine both together by asking the patient to press the chin downwards against the examiner's hand. Both muscles will, in normal circumstances, stand out and can be compared. Each sternomastoid may then be tested by asking the patient to rotate the chin to each side in turn against resistance; there will be weakness on moving the head way from the side of the impaired muscle.

Wasting of the trapezius can best be appreciated by inspection from behind; the power is tested by asking the patient to shrug the shoulders against resistance.

The hypoglossal (twelfth cranial) nerve

The tongue should be inspected for wasting and fasciculation indicative of a lesion of the lower motor neurone. The tongue

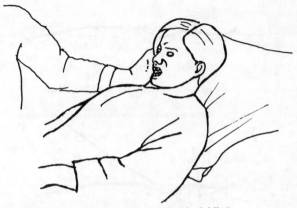

Fig. 37 Testing for meningeal irritation (neck rigidity).

should then be protruded; if there is unilateral weakness, it will deviate towards the paralysed side.

Supplementary tests

Under this heading are included tests which yield important information in special circumstances.

Meningeal irritation

Inflammation of the meninges due to infection or blood in the subarachnoid space evokes reflex spasm in the paravertebral muscles. In the cervical region this causes *neck rigidity* and painful restriction of passive flexion of the neck. If meningitis or subarachnoid haemorrhage is suspected, neck flexion should be tested with both hands behind the occiput of the supine patient (Fig. 37). The neck initially should be slowly flexed but in the early stages of a meningeal reaction, spasm may be more easily demonstrated if the neck is flexed abruptly. Normally the chin can be made to touch the chest without causing discomfort.

In the lumbar region passive movements of the lower limbs

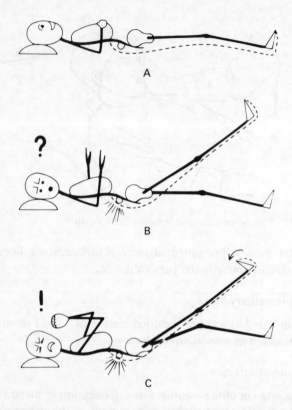

Fig. 38 Straight leg raising: A—patient lying supine is free from pain; B—straight leg raising is limited by tension of the root over the prolapsed disc causing pain; C—tension and pain are increased by dorsiflexion of the foot.

are restricted (*Kernig's sign*). The patient lies with one leg extended; the other leg flexed at the hip and knee. Keeping the hip flexed, the knee is then extended. When meningeal irritation is present, it will be impossible to extend the knee fully because of spasm in the hamstring muscles.

Nerve root irritation

When lumbar or sacral nerve roots are pressed upon, for example by a prolapsed intervertebral disc, stretching of the affected nerve may give rise to pain. For example, the sciatic nerve is tested by flexing the hip with the knee straight (*straight leg raising*) (Fig. 38). The leg is slowly raised and the patient is asked to report as soon as pain is experienced and to indicate the site of the pain. Normally 90° of painfree flexion of the hip should be possible.

THE DIAGNOSTIC PROCESS

Disturbance of function

The principal signs attributable to lesions of different components of the nervous system need to be understood and memorised.

Upper motor neurone (pyramidal tract) lesions cause (1) paresis or paralysis; (2) hypertonia of spasticity type; (3) increased tendon reflexes; (4) diminution or absence of abdominal reflexes; (5) an extensor plantar response.

Lower motor neurone lesions cause (1) paresis or paralysis; (2) hypotonia; (3) wasting; (4) diminished or absent tendon reflexes.

Cerebellar lesions. The main features are (1) ataxia; (2) intention tremor; (3) jerking nystagmus; (4) dysarthria of staccato or scanning type.

Generalised polyneuropathies cause (1) diminution of sensation affecting the distal aspect of limbs over 'stocking' and 'glove' distribution; (2) wasting and weakness of distal limb musculature; (3) loss of tendon reflexes.

Sensory tracts. Interruption of the *dorsal columns* causes (1) ataxia of gait and of limb movements aggravated by eye closure; (2) impaired position sense; (3) impaired vibration sense.

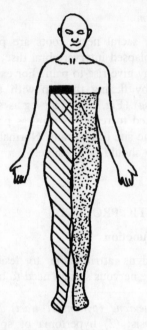

Fig. 39 Hemisection of the spinal cord (Brown-Sequard Syndrome). Ipsilateral loss of joint position sense (hatched area); contralateral loss of pain and temperature sense (dotted area).

Interruption of the *spinothalamic tracts* causes selective impairment of pain and temperature sensation.

Distribution of lesions

The identification of damaged neural structures is followed by the definition of the site or sites of their involvement.

1. A single lesion may affect diverse functions; for example, although hemisection of the spinal cord is a rare lesion, it is instructive to predict its effect from

study of Figure 26. Below the level of the lesion there will be ipsilateral upper motor neurone signs and loss of position and vibration sense (Fig. 39). There will also be contralateral loss of pain and temperature sense. At the level of the lesion there may be evidence of involvement of ipsilateral lower motor neurones.

2. Two or more discrete lesions may be defined, as for example, when an optic nerve lesion is found concurrently with evidence of spinal cord damage from multiple sclerosis.

3. Lesions may be systematised with similar types of fibres or cells being affected throughout the nervous system. A good example is motor neurone disease in which there is degeneration of upper and lower motor neurones in varying proportion at varying levels.

4. Diffuse damage also occurs as, for example, in neurosyphilis.

Pathological diagnosis

The diagnosis is incomplete until a pathological process has been identified. This involves considering the signs in the light of the history. Sudden neurological defects are usually vascular; a more chronic history of relapsing symptoms with anatomically unrelated physical signs may suggest demyelination. Chronic and progressive disorders suggest degenerative, metabolic or neoplastic pathologies.

If a patient with neurological disease is approached in this manner, it is often possible to make a firm diagnosis on clinical grounds alone though this may require confirmation by further investigation.

A summary of the basic examination of the nervous system is given on page 130.

6. The locomotor system

THE HISTORY

Pain and stiffness are the principal symptoms of lesions involving the locomotor system. Pain frequently has a characteristic pattern in relationship to physical activity. In rheumatoid arthritis, for example, pain and also stiffness are worst after a period of rest and gradually improve as the joints are used. In osteoarthrosis, in contrast, exercise makes the joint pain worse. While there is often a direct relationship to trauma, patients may incorrectly attribute their locomotor troubles to some antecedent injury.

The degree of functional disability can be assessed by asking questions such as, 'Can you dress yourself and how long does it take you to do so?' 'Can you walk to the shops?' and 'Do you have difficulty climbing up and down stairs?'

THE PHYSICAL EXAMINATION

The locomotor system includes joints, the muscles and the tendons which move the joints, and the bones and ligaments which provide support. Though any of these components can be affected by disease, joints are the most commonly disordered while muscles and tendons are rarely so. All are frequently involved by injury.

The locomotor system is examined by inspection and

palpation both at rest and in action. Nearly all of the structures are paired; every opportunity should be taken to compare an affected part with its normal counterpart. Such abnormalities as the restriction of joint movement, muscles wasting and injuries are particularly well suited to measurement and recording by diagram.

Inspection

This commences with observation of the patient's gait and posture and thereafter of joints, muscles and related structures.

Gait

The rhythm of the gait is often disturbed by pain. The patient takes the weight off the painful leg as quickly as possible and the timing is dot-dash, dot-dash, painful-normal, painful-normal. Painless loss or impairment of movement in a joint, as from bony or fibrous fusion, causes a contrary pattern of gait in that the long pause is on the abnormal leg. A waddling gait may be due to inadequacy of the gluteal muscles or to bilateral congenital dislocation of the hips. Characteristic gaits may also be of neurological origin, for example shuffling in parkinsonism.

Posture

This alters with age and disease particularly of the spine, e.g. kyphosis or scoliosis (p. 34); kyphosis in the thoracic region is a common abnormality in the elderly as a result of osteoporosis (deficiency of bone matrix) or occasionally of osteomalacia (demineralisation of bone).

Joints, muscles and related structures

Inspection of paired joints should compare the affected one with that of the other limb; minor swelling and other changes can thus be detected. The bulk and strength of the adjacent muscles should also be assessed because injury or disease of a joint is followed by muscle wasting, for example in the quadriceps femoris when the knee is involved. Active should precede passive movements, particularly if a painful lesion is present and the range through which the patient can move the joint should be measured. Passive movement need not be tested if active movement is unimpaired unless abnormal mobility is being sought.

Inspection of the locomotor system, like inspection of the skin, is often carried out piecemeal in the course of a physical examination. However, the locomotor system as a whole can be reviewed in the manner described below and illustrated in Figure 40. The required movements are facilitated if the examiner demonstrates what to do; at the same time this gives a range of movement for comparison.

The dorsum of the hands and wrists are first inspected. The patient is then asked to make a clenched fist, show the palms, touch the little finger with the thumb and put the wrists through a full range of movement. Inspection of the elbows is followed by asking the patient to bend, then straighten the elbows fully. The shoulder is then examined by raising the arms above the head, then touching first the back of the neck and thereafter the small of the back. In this way abduction, external rotation and internal rotation of the shoulder are tested in turn.

The neck is fully extended and flexed and the patient is requested to touch the tip of each shoulder with the ear to test lateral flexion and with the chin to test rotation. Forward flexion of the spine is tested by attempting to touch the toes with the knees straight, extension by leaning backwards, lateral flexion by sliding the hand as far as possible down the

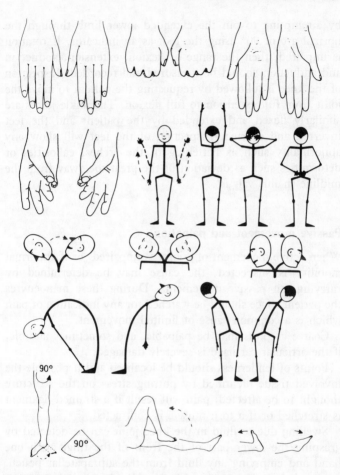

Fig. 40 Examination of active movements.

lateral side of the thigh and rotation by turning head and shoulders to the right and left. If forward flexion is full and painless, there is no need to test the other movements. Similarly if rotation of the hip is unimpaired, it is unlikely that other significant limitation is present. Rotation is measured by attempting to put the extended lower limb through the normal arc of 90° using the foot as an indicator. If rotation is impaired, then the range of flexion, extension, abduction and adduction should be measured and recorded. Inspection of the knee is followed by requesting the patient to move the joint from full extension to full flexion. The ankle joints are similarly flexed and extended by the patient and the feet inverted and everted. Inspection of the feet will show any abnormality such as flattening of the arches, callosities or deformities such as deviation of the great toe away from the midline (hallus valgus).

Passive movement and palpation

When active movement of a joint is impaired, or if abnormal mobility is suspected, the cause may be determined by carrying out passive movements. During these manoeuvres the patient's face should be watched for any indication of pain which is a common cause of limited movement.

Coarse crepitus may be palpable, and sometimes audible, if the articular cartilage is severely damaged.

Points of tenderness should be localised and if possible the involved tissue identified by putting stress on the structure thought to be affected; pain will result if a strained ligament is stretched or if a torn muscle is contracted.

Swelling due to fluid in the knee joint can be detected by grasping the lower part of the front of the thigh with one hand and emptying any fluid from the suprapatellar pouch. An attempt is then made with the other hand to depress the patella sharply onto the femur; a distinct tap indicates displacement of fluid and helps to distinguish the swelling from that due to synovial thickening.

The temperature of a swollen joint should also be compared by touch with that of the other limb.

Conclusion

Analysis of the history, followed by inspection, the assessment of limitation of movement, the localisation of the site of pain, the examination of any swelling as described on page 116, and specific tests of function of individual structures should enable a diagnosis to be made in most instances.

7. The integration of the physical examination

It is usual to learn first how to examine the major systems in turn as described in the preceding chapters of this book and every opportunity should be taken of obtaining practice both on student colleagues and on patients. When these methods have been mastered, the student must learn to integrate them so that the patient is subjected to as little inconvenience as possible. At the same time the routine must be flexible so that it can be readily adjusted according to the individual problem.

The evidence elicited in the course of the general examination is often the most highly significant of all the findings. It is available to the alert clinician from the moment of first contact with the patient even before the history taking commences. From the outset junior students should make a conscious effort to acquire this skill by observing all they can about the patient as they learn to examine each system in turn.

There is no correct sequence of performing a physical examination. The student must be prepared to modify and adapt until developing a method which is natural. Some clinicians examine patients from the feet upwards. Many doctors find the following a useful sequence, in which each stage should be initiated by inspection of the skin.

1. General examination of the patient.

This pays attention to such features as demeanour,

physique, gait, complexion, speech, intellect and mood. Weight and height should also be recorded and a specimen of urine tested for the presence or absence of protein, glucose, ketones, bilirubin, blood and urobilinogen. Other information such as the appearance of sputum and bedside charts, if available, must not be overlooked.

2. Feel radial pulse and examine hands and arms.

3. Examine head and neck.

4. Proceed now either to area mainly affected or to anterior chest (heart, lungs, breasts and axillae) and then to back (lungs and spine).

5. Examine abdomen, groins and male external genitalia.

6. Examine lower limbs.

7. Record blood pressure now, and again later if the patient is still not relaxed.

8. Ophthalmoscopic examination.

9. Rectal examination if indicated.

This is the sequence which will be followed in this chapter. An opportunity will also be taken of describing those methods of examination which have been mentioned only briefly elsewhere, including the inspection of the mouth and of the skin, the examination of a swelling and the use of the auriscope and the ophthalmoscope.

GENERAL EXAMINATION

Demeanour

Much may be learned from the patient's posture, dress and behaviour while the history is being recorded and from non-verbal communication as conveyed by eye-to-eye contact, facial expression, movements of the hands and other 'body language'.

Complexion

Normal colour of the face depends largely upon variations in skin blood flow and the amounts of melanin and haemoglobin present. The quantity of blood in the skin vessels and the haemoglobin level determine the reddish component. An excessive amount of reduced haemoglobin causes a purplish tinge (cyanosis).

Peripheral cyanosis occurs when an excessive amount of oxygen is extracted from the capillaries due to a low rate of blood flow and in a temperate climate the extremity affected will feel cold.

Central cyanosis is usually most obvious in the tongue and lips. It occurs when there is at least 4 gms of desaturated haemoglobin in arterial blood. It is commonly due to respiratory failure but also occurs in severe polycythemia and is caused by veno-arterial shunts (blue baby) or abnormal forms of haemoglobin such as methaemoglobin. In temperate climates it can be distinguished from peripheral cyanosis by the presence of warm extremities.

Melanin

Apart from race, increase in melanin results from sunlight, chronic inflammation in the skin, deposition of heavy metals especially iron, or over-production of melanocyte-stimulating hormone as in Addison's disease. Reduction in melanin results from lack of sunlight, hypopituitarism and enzyme deficiencies as in albinism.

Bilirubin

Jaundice is usually seen in the sclera and beneath the tongue before it is obvious in the skin. It may be overlooked if the patient is examined in artificial light.

Abnormal movements

Involuntary movements may be due to organic disease of the central nervous system. Their causes are discussed on page 65.

Abnormal sounds

Peculiarities of the voice may be characteristic; for example in myxoedema the voice is lowered in pitch and hoarse due to thickening of the vocal cords. A nasal quality of speech indicates a cleft palate or palatal paralysis, while disease of the larynx or damage to a recurrent laryngeal nerve lead to hoarseness or aphonia. The cry which is sometimes heard at the onset of an epileptic fit and stridor with laryngeal obstruction are further examples of abnormal sounds.

Abnormal odours

Examples include malodorous breath (halitosis) which may be associated with poor oral hygiene, ulcerative stomatitis or bronchiectasis. Very foul smelling eructations occur when there is a gastrocolic fistula bringing faecal contents into the stomach. The sweet smell of acetone in the breath in severe diabetic ketoacidosis is very obvious to some but not appreciated at all by others. A characteristic, rather sickly smell may occur in hepatic failure. A smell of alcohol should prompt the doctor to make enquiries about the patient's drinking habits.

Anthropometry and nutritional status

Routine examination should include the measurement of weight and height, without shoes, both for their immediate value and for future reference. Any recent change in weight must be regarded critically. An explanation for weight loss should be sought in terms of reduced intake and increased output of energy. Causes of reduced intake include loss of appetite and malabsorption. Increased energy loss occurs in hyperthyroidism, glycosuria, fever or a change to a more energetic lifestyle. Often there are combinations such as anorexia and fever in tuberculosis. A rapid gain in weight over a period of days is caused by fluid retention. This may occur premenstrually or indicate underlying disease, as in patients with cardiac failure.

Obesity can be assessed by measuring skin fold thickness with special calipers or by gently pinching a skin fold between thumb and finger.

The state of hydration

In all cases of salt and water depletion notably from vomiting, diarrhoea, sweating or polyuria, the state of hydration should be assessed by weighing if the previous weight is known. A dry tongue is apt to be deceptive as it may be due to mouth breathing. If, in an adult the blood pressure is low and the skin dry and inelastic, a major sodium and water deficiency state exists. Generalised oedema occurs if there is fluid over-load, as in cardiac failure, or hypoproteinaemia, as in the nephrotic syndrome.

Body temperature

The usual clinical practice is to measure axillary skin or sublingual temperature, the normal being 36.5–37.0°C. The rectal temperature is about 0.5°C higher. In accidental hypothermia special low-reading thermometer should be used.

The hands

Inspection

After the initial general appraisal of the patient, the specific physical examination begins with inspection of the hands.

Many people express themselves through their hands and indeed the dumb 'speak' through them. So also the thyrotoxic patient shows agitation (hyperkinesia) and the bereft, grief. Much can be learned about the patient from the appearance of the nails (e.g. well groomed or bitten) or of the fingers, ingrained with dirt or stained with tobacco. The number of observations of diagnostic value which can be made is vast and only a few examples are given:

Skin: spider telangiectases (p. 119) in cirrhosis of the liver.

Sclerae: bluish discolouration in iron deficiency and osteo-genesis imperfecta.

Subcutaneous tissue: tender areas in finger pulps from emboli in infective endocarditis (Osler's nodes).

Nails: splinter haemorrhages in infective endocarditis; flat-tening or 'spooning' (koilonychia) in iron deficiency; pitting in psoriasis.

Muscles: diffuse wasting and fasciculation in motor neurone disease.

Tendon: xanthomatous nodules in hypercholesterolaemia.

Joints: spindling of proximal interphalangeal joints in rheu-matoid arthritis.

Bones: osteophytes of terminal interphalangeal joints (Heberden's nodes) in osteoarthrosis.

Palpation of hands

The hot moist palm of hyperthyroidism contrasts with cold, rough skin of myxoedema.

Finger clubbing refers to a bulbous swelling of the terminal phalanges; it may also affect the toes. Clubbing is occasionally congenital but its development indicates serious disease of the lungs or heart and sometimes the gut or liver. In detecting the earlier stages, reliance is placed on flattening of the angle of insertion of the nails and fluctuation of the nail bases. The

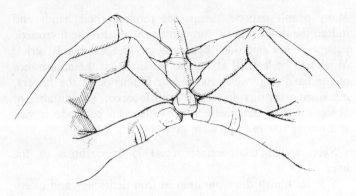

Fig. 41   Testing nail bed fluctuation for finger clubbing.

latter is tested by resting a suspected finger on the pulp of the examiner's thumbs while palpating the nail base with the forefingers, pressing first with one finger and then the other (Fig. 41). Fluctuation gives a floating sensation which is transferred from one finger to the other. A comparable technique is used for testing for fluctuation elsewhere (p. 118).

The upper limbs

The remainder of the upper limbs can next be examined, attention being paid particularly to dermatological, neurological or locomotor features as appropriate. One example is the painless subcutaneous nodules seen and felt over the upper ulna in some patients with rheumatoid disease.

The head

The patient's facial appearance may be pathognomonic of disease, for example the immobile stare of parkinsonism, the startled appearance of hyperthyroidism in a young person or the epicanthic folds in Down's syndrome. Attention has already been drawn to the transient facial expressions which may convey more important information than the patient's words.

The eyes, mouth and ears merit particular scrutiny.

The eyes. There may be an obvious abnormality seen from a distance such as swelling of the eyelids in myxoedema, proptosis and lid retraction in hyperthyroidism or ptosis affecting one or both eyes from various causes. For example a slight unilateral ptosis and a small pupil is indicative of a lesion of the cervical sympathetic nerves (Horner's syndrome). Closer inspection is also required in order to examine the eyelids, the ocular and palpebral conjunctiva (useful sites for checking clinical evidence of jaundice and anaemia), the iris and the pupil. Each of these structures may be involved in local disease or may show abnormalities pointing to a disorder elsewhere.

The mouth. Routine examination of the mouth must include inspection of the lips, tongue, teeth, gums, tonsils, palate, mucosa of the cheeks, floor of the mouth and the oropharynx. These can be seen easily and efficiently with the help of a spatula and a pocket torch. The colour of the mucosa gives a useful diagnostic clue to anaemia.

Carcinoma must be considered in the differential diagnosis of any chronic ulcer in or around the mouth; a characteristic feature is the hardness of the edge. A biopsy is essential when suspicion is aroused.

Cyanosis of the *tongue* is a good guide to central cyanosis (p. 106). Diffuse atrophy of the filiform papillae results in the smooth clean-looking tongue of iron or vitamin B_{12} deficiency. Excessive furring, by contrast, is of little diagnostic significance in spite of the concern it may cause.

The *teeth* are commonly affected by caries and they often become loose as the result of periodontitis and recession of the gums due to chronic gingivitis. These disorders may not only produce local symptoms but are also important as portals of entry for organisms causing infective endocarditis.

The *tonsils* enlarge to reach a maximum between the ages of 8 and 12 years, after which involution usually takes place. Failure to recognise this normal phase of lymphoid hyperplasia has, in the past, led to many unnecessary tonsillectomies.

The *oropharynx* can best be seen if the tongue is depressed with a spatula and the patient asked to say 'Ah' in order to elevate the soft palate. Pus from infection in the nose may sometimes be visible tracking down the back of the throat.

The ears

Auriscopic examination is indicated if there is earache or deafness. The pinna of the ear should be drawn gently upwards and backwards in order to straighten the external meatus and facilitate the insertion of the speculum of the auriscope (Fig. 42). The normal drum is pearly grey and a cone of reflected light is seen radiating at about 5 o'clock from the centre. In acute otitis media, the drum may be red, bulging and without a light reflex.

The neck

The neck should be inspected for any changes in the skin, scars, swellings, and arterial and venous pulsation. Systematic palpation should then be carried out with particular reference to any lymphadenopathy or enlargement of the thyroid gland (*goitre*). A goitre moves up on swallowing because the pretracheal fascia which envelops the thyroid gland is attached to the larynx. The principles involved in the examination of any

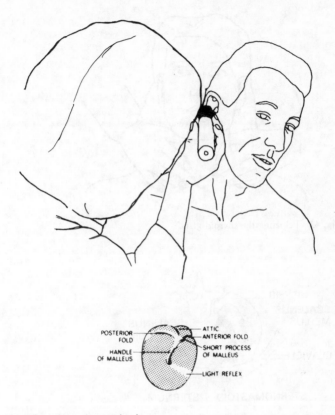

POSTERIOR FOLD
ATTIC
ANTERIOR FOLD
HANDLE OF MALLEUS
SHORT PROCESS OF MALLEUS
LIGHT REFLEX

Fig. 42 Auriscopic examination.

swelling (p. 3) apply to the assessment of a goitre. The patient should be sitting upright and the examination undertaken from behind (Fig. 43). Palpation for lymphadenopathy is carried out successively beneath the mandible, over the tonsillar lymph nodes, over the anterior and posterior triangles and above the clavicle. A site of particular importance, which is often overlooked, is behind the heads of the ster-

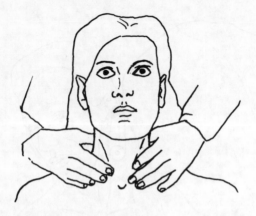

Fig. 43 Palpating the thyroid gland.

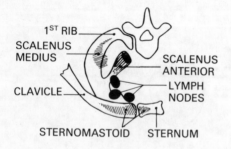

1ST RIB

SCALENUS MEDIUS

SCALENUS ANTERIOR

CLAVICLE

LYMPH NODES

STERNOMASTOID

STERNUM

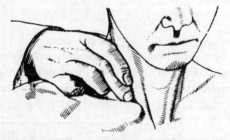

Fig. 44 Palpating the scalene lymph nodes.

nomastoids, where the scalene lymph nodes draining lesions in the chest or abdomen are frequently involved (Fig. 44).

Auscultation of the neck, over the great vessels, may reveal a bruit which in the absence of an aortic ejection murmur may indicate stenosis in a carotid or subclavian artery. A bruit heard over a goitre is indicative of increased vascularity of the thyroid gland and suggests hyperthyroidism.

Examination of the neck includes testing neck movements (p. 100), and assessing the XI cranial nerves (p. 92). It is completed from the front by feeling for the position of the trachea (p. 36) and inspecting the neck veins (p. 16).

The breasts

The breasts can readily be examined along with the chest and heart. Since the breast is the most common site of carcinoma

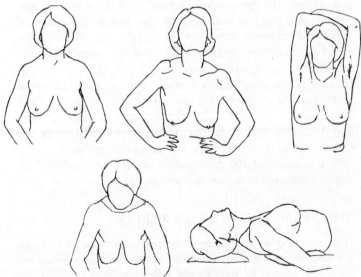

Fig. 45 Positions for examination of the breasts.

in women of all age groups, a general examination is incomplete unless both breasts have been examined (Fig. 45). Inspection for symmetry should be followed by palpation with the flat of the hand. Any mass must be regarded as a potentially malignant tumour. The axillae should also be examined for lymphadenopathy, the fingers of the right hand being used for the left axilla and vice versa (Fig. 46).

The trunk and lower limbs

Examination continues with that of the heart, chest, abdomen and spine and then with the lower limbs where the dermatological, peripheral vascular, locomotor and neurological components of the examination are integrated. It is worth re-emphasising that comparison of the two limbs greatly facilitates the examination. In the ambulant patient, pitting oedema can first be detected at the ankles by firm pressure for about five seconds. In the patient confined to bed, oedema is also sought over the sacrum and in the thighs. Evidence of venous thrombosis must not be overlooked (p. 29). Petechial haemorrhages, which may be the first manifestation of a haemorrhagic disorder, may be detected only in the legs because of the increased hydrostatic pressure if the patient is ambulant. After inspection and palpation along the lines indicated on page 99, the reflexes are assessed (p. 75), and thereafter other locomotor or neurological tests are carried out as determined by the individual problem.

When indicated the examination should be concluded by digital examination of the rectum (p. 58).

THE EXAMINATION OF A SWELLING

Any mass should be examined methodically in order to make a diagnosis and to plan the most appropriate investigations. Attention should be paid to the following features:

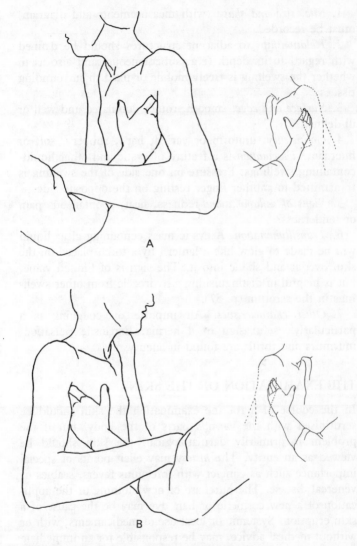

Fig. 46 A & B—palpating axillary lymph nodes.

1. *Site, size and shape* (with measurements and diagram) must be recorded.

2. *Relationships* to adjacent structures should be defined with regard to its depth (e.g. subcutaneous) and also as to whether the swelling is freely mobile or fixed to surrounding tissues.

3. *Surface and edge*: smooth, rough, lobulated and well or ill-defined?

4. *Consistency*: uniform or varied; hard, rubbery, soft or fluctuant? *Fluctuation* is a feature of cystic and other liquid-containing swellings. Pressure on one side of the swelling is transmitted to another finger resting on the opposite side.

5. *Signs of inflammation*: redness, heat, spontaneous pain or tenderness?

6. *Transillumination*. A cystic mass containing clear liquid will be made to glow like a lantern by a torch placed on the skin over it and shone into it. The sign is of limited value, but is helpful in distinguishing a hydrocele from other swellings in the scrotum (p. 57).

7. *Other characteristics*. An impulse on coughing is a particularly useful sign of a hernia. Expansile pulsation, murmurs and thrills are found in aneurysms.

THE EXAMINATION OF THE SKIN

In the course of a routine examination the skin should be scrutinised with the various parts of the body, but if the problem is primarily dermatological, the skin should be viewed as an entity. The *history* may elicit points of special importance such as contact with infectious fevers, scabies or venereal disease. The purchase of new clothing or the application of a new cosmetic or hair dye may be the cause of a skin eruption. Systemic or local use of medicaments, with or without medical advice, may be responsible for an immediate or delayed hypersensitivity reaction (urticaria or dermatitis).

Some skin lesions are manifestations of systemic disorders e.g. lupus erythematosus.

Physical examination

This consists largely of inspection supplemented by palpation to assess the texture of the skin, the consistency of a lesion and the local temperature.

Inspection of the skin will nearly always reveal some abnormality and any lesions present should be described. *Erythema* means reddening of the skin. A *macule* is a small circumscribed discoloration of the skin such as freckle. A *papule* is raised above the surrounding surface of the skin. A *vesicle* (blister) consists of liquid in the epidermis or the dermis; the larger variety is called a *bulla*. If the liquid within a vesicle becomes purulent, the lesion is known as a *pustule*. *Urticaria* is a raised pale area of skin caused by an increase in interstitial liquid surrounded by erythema due to capillary dilatation through an axon reflex. *Scaling* or *desquamation* is due to abnormal maturation of the skin and is particularly prominent in eczematous lesions and in psoriasis.

Examples of skin lesions

Purpura is due to spontaneous bleeding into the skin; the smallest lesions are known as petechiae and can readily be overlooked by the cursory observer. Their causes are manifold and range from a transient infection to serious disease such as leukaemia. *Spider telangiectases* consist of a central arterial dot from which radiate several dilated vessels, all of which can be obliterated by central pressure. Such spider naevi may occur in health and in pregnancy, but five or more suggests cirrhosis of the liver. In contrast, *Campbell de Morgan spots* are of no significance. They consist of small bright red or bluish haemangiomas especially on the trunk and are present, like seborrhoeic warts, in many elderly patients. They can be made paler by firm pressure conveniently applied by a pin head but can seldom be made to disappear because of the complexity of the dilated blood channels.

Puncture marks should raise suspicion of drug addiction. Linear markings known as *cutaneous striae* may be seen on the abdomen; those of recent origin are pink while older striae are whitish. They are due to stretching of the skin in obesity, from massive ascites or during pregnancy. In Cushing's disease or as result of high dosage adrenocorticosteroid treatment, purple striae appear over the pectoral regions and upper arms, the lower abdomen and upper thighs. Useful information may sometimes be gathered from examination of the *axillary and pubic hair*; for example, it is lost in hypopituitarism.

Benign *tumours* and primary or secondary malignant lesions occur in the skin and subcutaneous tissues. Examples of the former are *lipomas* and *neurofibromas*. *Basal cell carcinoma* (rodent ulcer) is a locally malignant tumour which is very frequently seen around the face in elderly persons. *Squamous cell carcinoma* (epithelioma), in contrast, is a rapidly growing tumour which may spread to adjacent tissues and the lymph nodes at an early stage. *Melanomas* (moles) may undergo malignant change and then rapidly disseminate to other organs. *Metastases* may occur in the skin from distant sites such as the lung or the breast and may be the first clinical manifestation of such a process. They usually consist of firm or hard nodules, less than a centimetre in diameter, which are often multiple.

Some lesions are indicative of important disease elsewhere; for example, *erythema nodosum*, which, as its name denotes is characterised by reddish swellings, occurs on the shins and is an allergic reaction to systemic disease, such as pulmonary sarcoidosis or a primary tuberculous infection. Lesions of apparently trivial significance such as acne should be taken

seriously as the disfigurement may constitute a social embarrassment and may have psychological repercussions.

THE USE OF THE OPHTHALMOSCOPE

The inspection of the fundi should be part of the routine
clinical examination. In different subjects, the colour and the
form of the visible structures will be seen to be as variable
as the facies. Familiarity with the range of normal appearances
is therefore essential. The acquisition of an ophthalmoscope,
like a stethoscope, is a necessity at an early stage in clinical
training. However it is advisable to learn to use the types
available before purchasing the instrument which suits best.
A model which has an interchangeable auriscope is particularly useful.

The ophthalmoscope contains a wheel carrying up to 30
lenses, arranged according to their focal length, which may be
placed in turn behind the hole in the mirror. The number of
each lens corresponds with its focal length expressed in
dioptres. A dioptre is the reciprocal of the focal length in
metres, e.g. 2 dioptres correspond to a focal length of half
a metre.

Convex (+) lenses bring the focal point nearer so that
anterior parts of the eye can be examined. They are essential
for obtaining a clear view of the fundus after removal of the
lens of the eye for cataract, or if the patient or the observer
is hypermetrophic (Fig. 47A). Concave (−) lenses are essential
if either is myopic. (Fig. 47B).

Technique in the use of the ophthalmoscope

Although most of the common lesions can be seen through
the untreated pupil, for a thorough examination of the fundus
the patient's pupil should be dilated by dropping a mydriatic
solution into the conjunctival sac. Tropicamide and cyclopen-

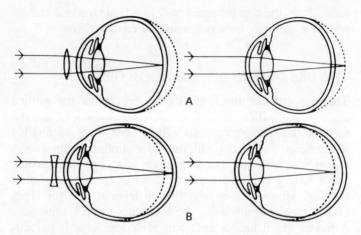

Fig. 47 Ophthalmoscopy: A—the hypermetropic (long-sighted) eye
B—the myopic (short-sighted) eye

tolate hydrochloride are preferred to homatropine as they act more rapidly and for shorter periods.

Attention to the following details of technique will enable the student to see the fundus without difficulty:

1. The environment should be darkened whenever possible.

2. The instrument should be held in the right hand with the forefinger on the lens adjustment wheel and the right eye used to look at the patient's right eye, and vice versa for the left eye. If the examiner has difficulty using the non-dominant eye, it is preferable to examine the patient from above (Fig. 48B).

3. The patient should be asked to look naturally, but not to stare, at some specific distant object. Blinking does not interfere with the view but does save the eye from watering. The eyelids should not be held open unless the patient is comatose or uncooperative.

4. If the examiner, for a reason other than astigmatism,

wears spectacles, these should be removed and an appropriate allowance made for the correction.

5. The examiner's face should be kept parallel to the patient's face. A common mistake is to look at right angles so that the operator's forehead or a lock of hair obliterates the view and the patient's gaze tends to wander (Fig. 48).

6. The examiner's eye should be kept as close as possible to the ophthalmoscope and the instrument should be held as near as possible to the patient's pupil without touching the eyelashes or cornea. The examiner's pupil, the holes in the head of the ophthalmoscope and in the mirror, and the patient's pupil make five small holes in a row; the closer they are the better the view.

7. Detailed examination is possible only if the instrument is steady. This is best achieved by resting the middle and ring fingers of the holding hand against the cheek of the patient.

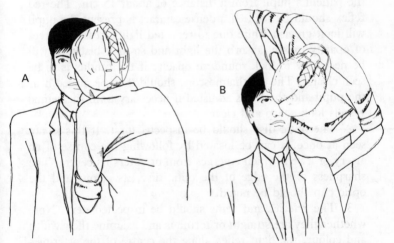

Fig. 48 Ophthalmoscopic techniques: A—the patient's gaze can be fixed on a distant point; B—using the right (dominant) eye to inspect the patient's left eye from above by an examiner who has difficulty in using the left eye. The patient's gaze is not obstructed.

8. It is important to look past the light reflected from the cornea and at the fundus beyond.

9. Considerate beginners and patients tend to hold their breath; this is unnecessary if the position described above is adopted.

10. The peripheral parts of the fundus are best seen by rotating the ophthalmoscope, and the examiner's head with it, so that the light is always on the pupil. Beginners tend to move the instrument up and down or from side to side; the light immediately leaves the pupil and they are left wondering why their glimpse of the fundus was so fleeting.

The routine inspection of the fundus oculi

The following procedure is advised:

1. With the setting at 'O' the light should be shone into the patient's pupil from a distance of about 15 cm. The red reflex should be seen. If a dense cataract is present the pupil will look greyish white due to reflected light. Lesser degrees of opacity mostly absorb the light and so look black. It will be necessary to look round an opacity if the fundus is to be seen clearly. The ophthalmoscope should then be placed near the pupil and the focus adjusted if necessary until the retinal vessels look sharp and clear.

2. The optic disc should be inspected first. If this is not seen at once, it can be located by following the course of an artery or a vein which emerges from or enters its centre. The sharpness of the edge of the optic disc, its colour and the optic cup should be noted.

3. The arteries and veins should be inspected next. Note whether they are straight or tortuous and examine their width and colour, the light reflex along the centre of the arterioles and the appearance at arteriovenous crossings. The artery usually crosses in front of the vein and blood columns should

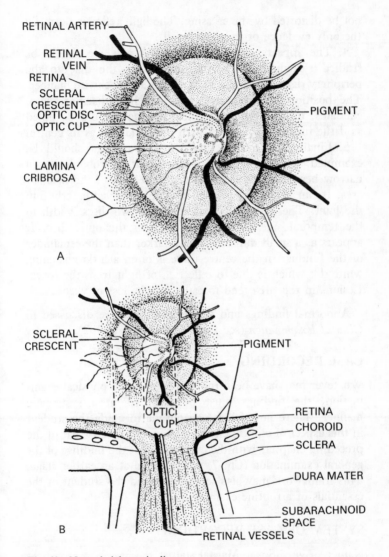

Fig. 49 Normal right optic disc.

not be distorted by the crossing. The light reflex is normally the only evidence of the vessel wall.

4. The appearance of the fundus as a whole should be studied systematically by radiating from the disc to the periphery right round in a clockwise or anticlockwise manner. The position of any abnormalities such as haemorrhages, exudates, or underlying choroidal changes should bᵥ noted as if the fundus was a clock with the optic disc as its centre.

5. Finally the macula and its surroundings should be examined. Unless the pupil is dilated, it is probable that a narrow beam will be required for inspection of the macular area. It can be seen at once if the patient looks directly into the light. The macula is situated about two discs' width to the temporal side of the lower pole of the optic disc. It appears as a small dull red patch, darker than the remainder of the fundus. In the centre there is often a little glistening white dot which is due to reflection of light from the fovea. Lesions in this area tend to cause serious loss of vision.

Abnormal findings and their significance are discussed in *Clinical Examination* (see Further Reading, p. 132).

CASE RECORDING

Whatever may have been the sequence of the physical examination, the findings must be recorded in a systematic manner. There now follows an outline to guide the student in this aspect of clinical clerking. The sequence is that of the preceding chapters with the exception that the findings of the general examination (Ch. 7) are recorded at an earlier stage. This framework may also serve to remind the student of the essentials of a routine examination.

SYSTEM OF CASE RECORDING

Name: Age: Sex: Marital status:
Address:

Occupation: (Where relevant state that of partner as well as patient).

Date of examination:

THE HISTORY

Present illness (p. 2)

Begin by naming the presenting symptoms and the duration of each. Proceed with a chronological account of the mode of onset and course of the illness up to the time of the interview.

Systematic enquiry

Record the presence or absence of cardinal symptoms such as cough, breathlessness, digestive or urinary troubles, pain, insomnia, or change in weight.

Drug history

Note any drugs taken and any *allergy*.

Previous health (p. 5)

Note any illness, operations, accidents, and their dates. Note any travel abroad.

Family history (p. 5)

Note age, health, or cause of death of parents, siblings, spouse and children.

Social and personal history (p. 5)

Record the relevant information about occupation, housing

and personal habits regarding recreation, physical exercise, alcohol and tobacco.

Psychological assessment (p. 6)

THE PHYSICAL EXAMINATION

General assessment (p. 105)

Height and weight should be noted.

In an introductory statement comment on the patient's demeanour and general condition, i.e. physique, nutrition, state of hydration, gait and posture.

Record any lesion of the skin or subcutaneous tissues or any finding (e.g. lymphadenopathy, goitre or finger clubbing) not recorded under a system heading.

Cardiovascular system

Arterial pulse and pressure (p. 14)

Rate, rhythm, wave form and volume of radial pulse. Blood pressure.

Venous pulse and pressure (p. 16)

Note height of the jugular venous pulse and waveform.

Heart (p. 19)

Character of apical impulse and position of apex beat and other pulsations; thrills.

First and second heart sounds; added sounds; murmurs.

Signs of cardiac failure.

Peripheral circulation (p. 26)

Peripheral pulses; skin temperature, colour and nutrition. Abnormal veins; signs of venous inflammation or occlusion.

Respiratory system

Note cough, character and quantity of sputum, cyanosis, wheeze or other respiratory difficulties.

Upper respiratory tract (p. 33)

Nose, tonsils, pharynx; trachea (p. 36)

Chest (p. 33)

Shape and lesions of chest wall; respiratory rate and depth. Note any abnormality found on palpation and percussion. Breath sounds, added sounds and vocal resonance.

Alimentary and Genito-urinary systems

Mouth (p. 111)

Lips, tongue, teeth, gums, buccal mucosa, tonsils, and palate.

Abdomen (p. 49)

Note any abnormality found on inspection, palpation, percussion or auscultation. (Diagrams are often helpful in recording these.)

External genitalia (p. 57)

Record any abnormality.

Rectum (p. 58)

Nervous system

Intellectual function (p. 8)

Speech (p. 62)

Cranial nerves (p. 81)

The principal features are:

Second (p. 81). Ophthalmoscopic examination; visual acuity; visual fields.

Third, fourth and sixth (p. 83). Eyelids (e.g. ptosis); pupils, size, shape, symmetry and reflexes; eye movements, diplopia and nystagmus.

Fifth (p. 87). Facial sensation, muscles of mastication.

Seventh (p. 89). Movements of facial muscles.

Eighth (p. 90). Hearing and auriscopic examination.

Tenth (p. 91). Phonation, movements of palate and posterior pharyngeal wall.

Eleventh (p. 92). Sternomastoid and trapezius muscles.

Twelfth (p. 92). Inspection of tongue and its movements.

Motor system (p. 63)

Inspection of muscles; involuntary movements; tone; clonus; power; coordination; gait; fine movements; dyspraxia.

Sensory system (p. 70)

Superficial touch and pain sensation; position and vibration sense; cortical sensory function.

Reflexes (p. 75)

Tendon, abdominal and plantar responses.

Supplementary tests (p. 92)

e.g. meningeal or nerve root irritation.

Locomotor system

Spine, limb joints, muscles, bones (p. 98)

Record any abnormality in these structures. Limitation of movement of any joint should be measured.

Urine (p. 104)

Test for glucose, blood and protein routinely and note any other abnormality discovered.

CLINICAL DIAGNOSIS

Tabulate either the differential diagnoses in order of probability and the various problems which the clinician must try to resolve.

FURTHER INVESTIGATIONS

Outline a plan of any further investigations considered necessary at this stage.

TREATMENT AND PROGRESS NOTES

These should be entered from day to day and must include the results of all investigations.

FINAL DIAGNOSIS

Analysis of data commonly leads to a single solution but there may be two or more and all should be recorded. Any unexplained facts should also be listed so that a summary of the patient's problems is readily available. This must be kept up to date as current problems are solved and new difficulties arise. The overall situation can then be reviewed by a glance at the summary, preferably kept on a special record sheet at the front of the patient's case notes.

CONCLUSION

It is salutary to remember that today's 'final diagnosis' may be inappropriate tomorrow because of further developments in the disease or as a result of new knowledge. The student must also keep in mind that, however complete the physical diagnosis may be, the individual patient may, as a result of the illness, still have to make considerable readjustments in family, social or occupational relationships. With some, physical rehabilitation may be a lengthy process, while others may have difficulty in coming to terms with the memory of an unpleasant illness or with the fear of its recurrence. What the student finds in hospital may indeed be just a prelude from the patient's viewpoint. This serves also as a reminder that this little book is only an introduction to much further study in relationship to the techniques of examination and to the significance of clinical data.

FURTHER READING

Macleod J, Munro J 1986 *Clinical Examination*, 7th edn. Churchill Livingstone, Edinburgh.

Index

133